MW00941020

Osteopathy and the Zombie Apocalypse:

Disaster survival with the masters of health, including alternative and natural medicine

Or

Why you want an OSTEOPATHIC medical doctor with you at the end of the world!

COPYRIGHT:
Mitchell A. Cohn, D.O.
Osteopathy and the Zombie Apocalypse – A Career Guide for Pre Med and Pre-College Students
Publisher: Mitchell A. Cohn, D.O.

© 2012, Mitchell A. Cohn, D.O.
Contact: Dr.Cohn@itsallconnected.net

DISCLAIMER:

All of the information in this book is based upon the author's personal experiences, readings, treatment by, and dealings with MD's, DO's, DC's, Acupuncturists, traditional Chinese medicine practitioners, various other medical professionals, and acrobats - most of whom he has worked with and been treated by over the past 50 years or more – except the acrobats.

Nothing in this book should be construed as medical advice. If you have healthcare concerns, you should seek advice, diagnosis, and treatment from a qualified medical professional, especially, if you learn anything at all from this book – a qualified osteopathic physician.

MISSION:

Having been an osteopathic physician and surgeon for more than 25 years who practices primarily hands-on diagnosis and manipulative medicine, I bring a different viewpoint regarding healthcare than your average doctor. While accepting and practicing the art and science of western medicine, in its entirety, I also bring to patients, healthcare providers, and healthcare organizations a message that there is a great deal more to healthcare than is currently offered by most practitioners and facilities. There are other dimensions to health including not just the physical, but also the emotional, cultural, and spiritual dimensions.

Specifically, I am concerned about the replacement of human touch, caring, and the supplanting of human intelligence and intuition by technology. This loss to healthcare quality and integrity must be recaptured in this age of tremendous technological advancement which has actually resulted in a decline of American well-being. It is through human touch and re-introduction of humanity into medicine that advancements in healthcare will be made, not just through technological innovation.

If this book is meant to accomplish anything, it is
- to broaden awareness of osteopathic medicine, principles, and practice;
- to get more patients to demand and expect appropriate personalized care;
- to make more patients aware that there are more complete alternatives to either MD-type or chiropractic-type care, especially when it comes to the treatment of pain;
- to get more providers and healthcare facilities to incorporate osteopathic manual diagnostics and treatment into their practices;
- to interest more premedical students, existing osteopathic students, and even existing physicians and

other providers in learning more about osteopathic principles and manual medicine and incorporating it into their practices;

- and to return medicine to its roots of humanity and human touch which do more to help people get better than technology will ever do by itself.

REAL LIFE:

One day, as I was walking up the steps to my dentist's office, I received a call. Without exaggeration, the woman on the line sounded desperate.

"Doctor, I've had pain in my chest for nearly four months. I've had every test known to man and still the doctors have found nothing. I've been to my own doctor, the lung doctor, and the cardiologist. The pain is horrible. I'm at my wits' end. Today they took blood to run nearly a hundred tests. If they don't find anything, I don't know what I'll do."

I said, "Ma'am. Can I ask you a couple of questions? Is the pain sharp, burning, dull, or pressure-like?"

"Sharp," she said. "Very sharp."

"Does it ever go away? When you rest, for instance?"

"Not really. No."

I had an idea what was going on. "I see," I continued. "Does it hurt in front or in back or both?"

"Both," she answered.

"Mmm hmm. And does it hurt when you take a deep breath all the way in?"

"Oh, YES!" she exclaimed. "Terrible, just terrible."

"Does it hurt when you exhale all the way?"

"Oh, YES!"

"Ma'am," I said, "I suspect you have a rib out of whack. Why don't you come in at 2:30 tomorrow afternoon and I'll see what we can do. If I'm wrong, you've lost nothing. If I'm right, your pain should resolve quickly."

"Oh, THANK YOU!" she said. "I'll be there."

The next morning, however, I got a call: "Doctor, I'm afraid I'll have to cancel our appointment, today."

"Oh?" I asked, "Why?"

(I'm actually quoting her, here.) "Well, she said, "Those blood tests came back and one of them was slightly off. I want to go to the cardiologist before we go any further."

"I see," I said. "Before you decide, I'd like to point out two things, though. First, nobody's blood tests are perfect all the time. At any given moment, there will be slight variations and slight deviations from normal. If you take a hundred blood tests, it is likely that at least one or two at any given minute will fall slightly outside the 'normal' range.

Second, you can still see the cardiologist, but it makes sense to come in for diagnosis and possible treatment. It's all non-invasive and won't hurt you. If we fix it, your troubles are over. If we don't, you can still continue with the cardiologist and have all the tests or treatments he recommends."

"No. No. I'm going to see the cardiologist. Thank you, anyway."

I never did see that lady.

But, that's not the end of the story. There is a more interesting moral.

I went home, saddened but bemused. I have four children. At the time, my oldest was about 16 and my youngest was 7. I told them each the story, individually, without telling them what I thought was going on and asked them what they thought.

When I told my daughter, the oldest, she said, "She's got a rib out of place." I smiled.

Throughout the evening, I went down the line and asked each of my three boys what they thought about the story. Right down to my 7 year old, they each said, "She's got a rib out of whack."

This is the moral: Why couldn't this woman's doctors make that diagnosis when even a child could do it?

The answer lies within this book.

Conventions Adopted for Writing this Book:

Definitions and conventions for writing this book:

- MD:

    Allopath or Allopathic physician; medical doctor trained at a standard, non-osteopathic medical school

- DO:

    Doctor of Osteopathic Medicine, aka Doctor of Osteopathy = Osteopath (not to be confused with foreign osteopaths who are not physicians), Osteopathic doctor, osteopathic physician; Medical Doctor trained at an American osteopathic medical school

- DC:

    Doctor of Chiropractic or Chiropractic Medicine = chiropractor; Chiropractic physician trained at a chiropractic medical school

- "He"/ "She":

    will be interchangeable so as not to offend any gender

- OMM = OMT:

    Osteopathic Manipulation, Osteopathic Manipulative Medicine, and Osteopathic Manipulative Treatment or Osteopathic Manipulative Therapy ; all refer to the methods of using one's hands to diagnose and treat patients by applying specific forces to specific body parts to effect a specific health-related outcome. All of these terms will be used interchangeably in this book.

- Case Studies:
    > In any of the anecdotes or case studies presented, all of which are true and accurate, only the details which might lead to identifying the patient or person involved have been changed in order to protect the person's privacy.

Shooting for Average:

In this book, I will be writing about what the AVERAGE MD is taught vs. what the AVERAGE DO is taught vs. what the AVERAGE DC (chiropractor) is taught – as well as what their licenses generally allow them to do (not that licenses matter in an apocalyptic situation!)

Some MD's have better diagnostic skills than others and almost certainly better than some DO's. Some have knowledge of natural medicine, and a very, very few have studied manual medicine techniques. Not every single MD is dependent on technology for their diagnoses or their treatments ... but the VAST MAJORITY ARE DEPENDENT ON TECHNOLOGY FOR ALL ASPECTS OF DIAGNOSIS AND EVEN MORESO FOR ALL ASPECTS OF TREATMENT.

To some extent, the same is true for chiropractors (with exceptions): I've never been to a chiropractor who wasn't reliant to a greater or lesser extent on x-ray findings and who didn't require x-rays before they would consider treating a patient.

On the other hand, some DC's do learn more than just spinal manipulation. Some know a great deal about medicinal treatments and laboratory diagnostics. Many know about natural treatments. Some have learned other types of manipulation including muscle energy or emphasize unusual treatments such as Atlantoaxial treatment. Some learn whole body manipulation, though from my experience, a majority does not. Some have even learned surgery, though with rare exception, they're generally not allowed to use it. Again, I have to restrict my writing to what the AVERAGE DC is taught and/or practices.

Osteopathic education tends to emphasize "people skills" and listening to our patients. Although some MD's are naturally gifted listeners and some may be taught the skill by individual mentors, as a profession this is not the most valued skill. I, in fact, patterned my own listening and people skills after a very fine MD, Dr. Sidney Prystowski*, of Detroit, not a DO, per se. Throughout my osteopathic education, however, people skills, relating to patients, and really listening to them were always highly emphasized. We osteopathic students were inculcated with the mantra, "85% of all diagnoses come from a good history," – i.e. the vast majority of diagnoses can be made by LISTENING to the patient.

In addition, osteopathic physicians have traditionally been taught that most of the remaining diagnoses can be made by employing well-honed physical diagnostic skills – from the well-known 'looking in the eyes and ears' of a patient and listening to their hearts and lungs, to far more sophisticated palpatory diagnostic skills (diagnosing by using our sense of touch).
When was the last time your MD actually touched you?

As osteopathic students were taught to use our skills and our intelligence to make diagnoses – and to use technological tests such as x-ray, MRI, EMG, blood tests, etc. to confirm, differentiate, or hone our diagnoses – not to make the diagnoses for us.

D.O.'s – whether we use all our skills or not in today's technologically-driven healthcare, are each taught ALL of the physical diagnostic, technological diagnostic, and treatment skills available in western medicine, with emphasis on listening/history-taking, physical diagnosis skills, manual diagnostics, medicinal prescription, surgery, and virtually every other type of available medical care.

The addition of plant medicinals and naturopathy is a skill lacking in all fields of medicine except naturopaths, though a much higher percentage of D.O.'s than M.D.'s generally take it upon themselves to learn about nutritional supplementation and natural remedies.

So, despite the widely varying knowledge and practices of individual practitioners, this book will emphasize what the average student within each profession is likely to encounter during their respective educations.

*In doing research for writing this book, sadly, I learned that Dr. Prystowski died at the age of 93, only four months before the book was completed.

INTRODUCTION:

I AM NOT A BIGOT!

It seems like an odd thing to say, but I am certain to be accused of bigotry against the other major health professions. This is because I make no attempt at political correctness which would require me to water down the information I have to impart.

I want to be absolutely clear because I don't want to get angry emails and letters from people whose experiences differ – or whose father, mother, aunt, brother or other relative, family friend, or erstwhile acquaintance happens to be a medical practitioner other than an Osteopathic Physician: I harbor no personal prejudices against any group. I and my family have had both terrible treatment and superb treatment by numerous members of each profession. There are wonderful MD's and very poor MD's, good chiropractors and bad chiropractors, good DO's and bad DO's. This is true of any profession. As I always say, what do you call a doctor who graduates at the bottom of his class? … Doctor.

With this said, it must be understood that there are limitations in knowledge within all professions – though I tend to find Osteopathic Doctors have a far broader training than the other recognized medical professions. In reality, there are also limitations in the practices legally allowed within each state, though the laws differ from state to state. In particular, even if a chiropractor is taught far more than just chiropractic manipulation of the spine and may be capable of doing much more than that in the extreme survivalist situation, in real life, in most states, he is legally prohibited from doing surgery and prescribing medicines, even if he knows how to do it. I also acknowledge that due to their medical philosophy – many, if not most – would not even want to perform such treatments.

It should also be noted that there are a very tiny minority of MD's who have gone far beyond their initial training to study areas of medicine such as herbal and naturopathic remedies, prolotherapy, and even osteopathic manipulation. This is not the norm, however.

I have also known chiropractors who have gone back to medical school to become a DO or an MD. I know of others who never did so, but have expressed the wish that they had.

It is also an unfortunate truth that the majority of DO's actually practice only allopathic-style medicine[1] – a loss for their patients and a loss for our profession. We'll examine why this is, later in the book. Others, though, specialize in Osteopathic Manipulative Medicine (OMM). This is not, however, the ideal. The ideal osteopathic medical practice would incorporate ALL forms of good and effective treatment within a single physician and her practice. It is my hope that this book will convince some of you to not only enter into osteopathic medicine as a career, but to understand the importance of the role of quintessentially osteopathic knowledge and hands-on skills that will separate you from the pack and make you, truly, the ELITE, COMPLETE PHYSICIAN you were meant to be.

You should also be aware that DO's make up a growing portion of the medical community with each passing year. When I graduated osteopathic medical school in 1986, there were only about 24,000 DO's, comprising only about 4% of all U.S. physicians. At that time, there also only 15 osteopathic medical schools. As of this writing, the number of DO's in the US has tripled to well over 70,000 who now comprise approximately 7% of all US physicians.[1] The number of osteopathic colleges has also more than doubled to 32.[2] This means that osteopathic influence is growing within the medical field and every one of you who chooses to become a DO can have a tremendous impact on the direction our profession will go as we grow, in the future.

[1]Allopathy refers to the type of medicine more commonly known as 'conventional western medicine.' It is a system of medical diagnosis and treatment which is based upon the use of pharmacologic agents which generally have the opposite effect of the symptom or problem being treated. For example, if a patient has a stuffy nose due to swelling of the linings of the nasal passages, the patient is given a medication, known

as a decongestant, which has the action of reducing the swelling, thereby opening up the nasal passages. In addition, allopathy encompasses the use of surgical treatments. Moreover, allopathy appears to emphasize the diagnosis and treatments of the separate systems of the body.

Allopathy is a term frequently used by non-MD or non-conventional healthcare providers. The term is, however, generally rejected by MD's who consider it either pejorative or unnecessary; unnecessary because this style of medicine is practiced by the majority of western physicians and, in their opinions is the only true practice of 'medicine.'

Of course, this makes no sense because there are a wide variety of other forms of 'medicine' practice including Traditional Chinese Medicine, various forms of acupuncture, Ayurvedic medicine, homeopathic medicine, and naturopathic medicine, to name just a few. It can safely be said that these forms of medicine, which MD's refer to as 'alternative' or 'complementary' are actually practiced as the primary form of treatment by billions of people around the world, and as a secondary form of medicine by many, many more.

For this reason, it makes sense to have a simple word we can use to specifically refer to 'western conventional medicine.' No offense is intended by the use of the word in this book. It is simply a useful term to distinguish Allopathy or "Allopathic-style" medicine (the use of primarily pharmacologic agents and surgery, as described above) from other forms of medical including Osteopathic Medicine which, in fact, incorporates all allopathic modes of treatment. Osteopathic medicine, is separated from the straight practice of allopathy, however, by the addition of manual (hands-on) diagnostics and treatment as well as a unique philosophy regarding the patient not only as a series of systems which must be treated and kept healthy, but as a unit which encompasses the physical, mental, and spiritual well-being of the individual. Of course, some MD's will naturally incorporate such philosophies (one is mentioned below), but such a philosophy does not exemplify allopathic medicine, is not taught at most MD medical schools, and is definitely not part of the overall philosophy of allopathic medical care.

† If, at any time, a reader can demonstrate that any statements in this book are incorrect or based upon misinformation or misunderstanding, especially of the other professions, I welcome the education and will make appropriate corrections in future editions.

WHY ARE YOU READING THIS BOOK?

In short: to learn that you have a choice.

If you've ever needed a doctor, most likely you believed that your only real choice was to seek the services of an MD. Some of you have probably also sought the services of chiropractors. Others may have thought, "Well, there really isn't any difference between seeing a doctor, a nurse practitioner (NP), or a physician's assistant (PA)."

To some extent, as regards allopathic medicine, you would be right: in many ways, there is little difference between what an NP or PA does and what an MD does, depending upon the MD's area of practice. Most NP's can even have independent practices and do pretty much what any family practice MD does. I know this will offend some of my allopathic colleagues, but I'm afraid it's quite true. NP's can treat patients with colds and take care of basic health maintenance, order diagnostic tests, and prescribe medicines.

Many of these things a chiropractor cannot do – and in most cases – claim they would not want to. It doesn't fit with the chiropractic philosophy. They are generally taught to treat the spine, improve nerve function, exercise, eat healthily, and the rest will take care of itself. In many ways, I freely admit, they are not wrong. This focus on 'prevention' is actually also very much part of the osteopathic philosophy.

An MD, NP, or PA, of course, is also taught that things like exercise and eating healthily is essential to good health. They are not, however, taught anything about the spine or how to fix it, unless it is truly 'broken' in some way measurable by x-rays, MRIs, or technological studies performed by sticking needles into muscles and nerves to measure electrical activity in these tissues. I will say this about such needle studies:

OUCH!

Outside of the basics which NPs and PAs, are taught, however, an MD is actually trained to do much more and to think in far more expansive ways which are vital to diagnosis and treatment, especially of health problems which don't fit neatly into common, daily seen illnesses or disorders. At the risk of offending NPs and Ps – and I speak from much experience in dealing with these groups – their views, their knowledge, and their expertise in dealing with complex problems are often very limited. It is for these reasons that NPs must have working agreements with supervising physicians and PAs may not work independently of a physician, at all.

In addition, specialist MD's can do all kinds of things that NPs and PAs can't. Surgery, for one. Becoming a radiologist, cardiac interventionist, brain surgeon, etc. Those doors are closed to anyone who isn't an MD.

Or are they?

What if you had the chance to be under the care of a professional who knows EVERYTHING an MD, NP, or PA knows … and EVERYTHING a chiropractor knows (and much more, in terms of hands-on treatment which chiropractors don't know) … and who can make diagnoses without being completely reliant on technology to do the work for them … and who can actually make people BETTER – not just make them feel better, but actually make them healthier … in ways which none of the other professions or paraprofessions can do? What if this professional, like an MD, had no limits to what he can do or what kind of medicine he can practice?

What if there was some kind of physician who actually knows more about the body than your average MD? What if his training in that type of medicine could allow him to do amazing things most MDs could never dream of doing? What if he could understand not only how each organ system acts, how it interacts with other organ systems, even how it affects the nerves, muscles, and skeletal systems – and how to improve how those organs function without using any medicines or fancy technology?

YET ... he would also have at his disposal every diagnostic tool, instrument, and technology, every treatment, every medicine, every surgery which an MD has. What if the difference between this other Doctor and an MD was simply ... he has more diagnostic and treatment tools and knowledge of the body's workings, and knows when it's best to use those tools and when it's best to use other methods of treatment, medication, and technology? Wouldn't that make him a more *complete* physician? Wouldn't it put him in a league of his own?

This physician has a name. His/her name is "Doctor of Osteopathic Medicine." – DO.

That is why I call DOs 'Elite, Complete Physicians.'

Let me tell you two brief stories, both of which are true, involving people I have come to know through my osteopathic medical career.

First, is a brief story about an MD., a neurologist, who jokingly refers to himself as an "MD gone bad." He found that as an MD neurologist, all he could do for his patients was offer them medicine to hide their symptoms – never cure them -- or he could refer his patients to a neurosurgeon and pray the patient got better after being sliced open and having their innards rearranged and/or parts removed, and suffering, in many cases, a long recovery time. Worse, many patients, especially ones who underwent some kinds of back surgery would not only never improve but, would be worse off and in more pain than before the surgery. Moreover, in many cases, he knew that once the surgery was done, the patients' anatomy was forever changed. After that, any effort to undo the surgically-induced damage would most likely be ineffective and result in even further damage.

This wise and compassionate MD said, in essence, "I can't really help these people get better. Isn't there something I can learn to do that will actually help them and maybe even cure them?"

That's when he discovered Osteopathic Manipulation. He took all the post-graduate courses he could in OMM. He studied diligently and practiced. It took years of additional work, but he became an amazing practitioner of the art and science of osteopathic manipulative medicine.

And he never looked back. He even went on to teach OSTEOPATHIC students the ins and outs of OMT.

The second story is about a nurse. He was an RN who got sick of what he saw going on in medical practice: all the unnecessary drugs, the surgeries, and people just not getting better. After years as a nurse, he decided he wanted something different – a way to really help people without all that 'garbage.' He went back to school … and became chiropractor.

Now, you would think that someone who has gone through that much schooling would have felt he made a wise decision and stuck with it. After years as a chiropractor, however, he became disillusioned. Again, he saw the failings of a limited system of practice. While chiropractic could work wonders for some problems, it could do nothing at all for others. In fact, by his state's law, he was limited to treating the spine, even when manipulation of other body areas might be beneficial. Moreover, he apparently came to the conclusion that not all drugs are bad and not all surgeries are useless.

Guess what this crazy man did?

That's right, he decided to go back to school, once again, to become a Doctor of Osteopathic Medicine, so that all tools, and all methods of diagnosis and treatment would be available to him.

As a quick side-note: I actually recently met a chiropractor who took a different route: As a chiropractor, he felt limited, but rather than go through four more years of medical school and two or more years of residency training, he went back to get his RN degree – and get his Nurse Practitioner license. That way, he could do the things that MD's could do ... and could still do manipulation to help his patients.

I give all of these doctors credit for realizing the shortcomings in their training. I definitely credit them for being inventive in meeting their desires and for having the fortitude to return to school when they were well into their 40's or older.

On the other hand, wouldn't it have made more sense just to become an osteopathic doctor, *in the first place?*

WHO AM I AND WHY SHOULD YOU LISTEN TO ME?

For starters, I once wanted to be an MD. I also thought that was my only choice if I wanted to become a full-fledged doctor. I had excellent grades. In fact, I was third in my high school senior class of over 620 students. I took nearly all of the Advanced Placement classes available while in high school and started college at this little-known school, the University of Michigan, in Ann Arbor, as a sophomore rather than as a freshman. In other words, I wasn't exactly an academic disgrace.

When it came time to start looking into applying to medical schools, though, I wasn't sure what to do or where to apply. One day, I walked into the university's career center, and while waiting for my appointment with the counselor, I looked around. That's when I had the great, good misfortune that would change the course of my life forever.

Career counseling centers have dozens of seemingly useless throw away pamphlets and brochures scattered all about. I found myself standing in front of a carrousel of such pamphlets. Most were about becoming a doctor or a nurse or such, but one caught my eye. It talked about something I'd never heard of before. It was called Osteopathic Medicine. I read it while I waited.

You mean I can be doctor who can fix people with his hands?? Wow. That blew me away. I couldn't say why, at the time, but everything I read about osteopathic philosophy – holism, treating the patient as more than an object or a disease, the way the body parts worked together and could be moved in such a way that the body could heal itself, if we just opened up the blood and nerve pathways – it all just intuitively made sense to me. And I could still prescribe medicines and do surgeries, if I thought it was called for.

Unfortunately, some people, including my family doctor, Sidney Prystowski, MD, tried to talk me out of applying to osteopathic school. Dr. Prystowski's reasoning seemed sound enough, but it didn't feel right. He told me, "There's nothing wrong with being an osteopath, but you'll have a hard time getting privileges to work at MD hospitals."

But what about that other stuff I could learn that you don't learn in MD schools??

Well, I admit I didn't apply to osteopathic colleges that first year, but my heart wasn't at all in the process. Needless to say, I was not accepted into medical school.

The next year, I said, "Screw it! I'm going to apply to the osteopathic colleges out there. I don't care what anybody says!"

Just as a safety net, though, I applied to an MD school – the American-run medical school on the island of Grenada. I figured, "What the heck. If I don't get into osteopathic school, which is what I really want, at least I could go to school in a tropical paradise."

And, so it went; I was accepted to the medical school on Grenada.

A few weeks later, I had the most interesting interview at some school in distant Des Moines, Iowa. It was a far cry from a grueling, truly heartless, anger-inducing interview I had previously at an MD school.

That previous MD school interview started with the interviewer, an MD, going through 20 pages of essays I'd had to write for my application. He'd marked up my essays and made numerous notations and squiggles and arrows. He made me feel like I was in the hot-seat in a police interrogation. He fired questions at me left and right. He told me to explain this answer and that. He found that this answer to question 18 conflicted with that answer in question 2. "Explain how you reconcile that," I was ordered.

I calmly answered all of his questions, and many new ones he threw at me. When I walked out, I felt like I'd just come through a war. If that was what med school was like, DAMN! I didn't want to go through that. I was sure I had failed the interview miserably.

As it turned out, an admissions counselor later told me that I'd received the highest recommendation for admission into that MD school that my interviewer had ever given anyone.

So WHAT?! That's not the way I wanted to spend my life, among people like that.

The interview at the osteopathic college in Des Moines, however, was the polar opposite. I was actually even more worried, having been through that prior interview and knowing that in Des Moines, I would be interviewed by not one, but three, interviewers, simultaneously.

Nervous, I walked into the office where the interview was to take place and low and behold ... I saw Colonel Sanders, all 6-plus feet long of him leaning back in his chair with his feet up on his desk. The other two interviewers were missing. In his big, basso profundo voice, the Colonel look-alike drawled, "They'll be back, soon. They had to take care of some, ah, physiologic functions," and he smiled.

The interview was an amazing experience. They wanted to know about ME, not about my achievements, or my grades, or my prior schooling. In fact, I was prepared to explain away a 'D' I'd gotten in biochemistry (because it was a self-taught class and I started the class half-way through the term, against my professor's better judgment – the professor had been right) – but the interviewers weren't interested in my D. The Colonel said, "It happens." They wanted to know my personal philosophy and whether I thought I would be a good doctor and why. They wanted to know who *I* was.

I learned it's not just what you know, but who you are that truly determines whether you will be a good doctor; a good osteopathic physician.

I walked out of the interview, all smiles, literally knowing they were going to accept me. And it was a good thing, too, as you'll see shortly.

And guess what? Dr. Prystowski may have been right at the time, but in the many years since our encounter, osteopathic physicians have been accepted onto staffs of virtually every hospital in the country and practice everywhere medicine is practiced. The distinctions between DO's and MD's have shrunk to the point that most patients not only don't know the difference between MD's and DO's, but many who have osteopathic doctors are not even aware that their doctor isn't an MD.

In some ways, that's nice, meaning DO's are completely accepted. Yet in some ways, that's not necessarily such a great thing, but only because so many DOs practice just allopathic-style medicine.

I have discovered over the years that, of those patients who are aware of the "D.O. difference" and have EXPERIENCED the difference of true osteopathic care, MANY say they'd either preferentially seek out a D.O. or would NEVER go to an M.D., again. While perhaps a bit extreme (even I go to MD specialists, when necessary), the sentiment is appreciated – and should be noted by my allopathic-style osteopathic colleagues.

Okay, SO? What does any of this have to do with surviving the Zombie apocalypse?

Compare this 'Zombie Survival' question to the standard question: "If you were stranded on a desert island, what one medicine/tool/person, etc. would you want with you? (Personally, I'd want a working satellite phone with built-in GPS – unless the world had gone to Hell, in which case I'd prefer a very attractive, intelligent, healthy, kind, and subservient mate well-versed in survivalist techniques!)

IT'S PERSONAL

Grenada: The invasion commenced at 05:00 on October 25, 1983. I was in my second year of medical school. Had I not gone to school at the University of Osteopathic Medicine and Health Sciences (now, the Des'Moines College of Osteopathic Medicine), I would still have been in my second year of medical school – on Grenada.

"The Invasion of Grenada, codenamed **Operation Urgent Fury**, was a 1983 United States-led invasion of Grenada, a Caribbean island nation with a population of about 91,000 located 100 miles (160 km) north of Venezuela. Triggered by a bloody military coup which had ousted a four-year revolutionary government, the invasion resulted in a restoration of constitutional government."

"After a 1983 internal power struggle ended with the deposition and murder of revolutionary Prime Minister Maurice Bishop, the invasion began on 25 October 1983, less than 48 hours after the bombing of the U.S. Marine barracks in Beirut."[3]

The American medical students had been held at the island's medical facility.

Disaster makes you think.

My desire to become someone who could help people even in a disaster, with virtually nothing but my hands and whatever I could scrounge, actually goes back further than the short-lived war in Grenada.

Alas, Babylon, a book about surviving nuclear war, made me think, too. I read the book in elementary school. When I was a kid, we weren't as over-protective of our children as people are, today. Adults of that era apparently believed that since we children lived every day of our lives with the threat of nuclear war, perhaps we should confront our fears. Perhaps we should learn that disaster, even global nuclear war, despite its terrors and hardships, may be survivable.

Ever since reading Alas, Babylon, the thought always went through my mind: what could I do for a career that, in the event of global disaster, would still make me useful?

The month after the invasion of Grenada and the rescue of the American medical students, the soon-to-be-Emmy-winning landmark made-for-TV movie, The Day After was released on November 20, 1983. The movie was based upon the reality of all the science known and accepted at that time. I remember being riveted to the TV, watching with all my being and intensity (probably when I should have been studying my medical books, as it was a Sunday night). Afterward, there were news discussions held and for some time thereafter, there were political discussions and debate. It seems to me, though, it was all for naught when only a year or so later, I became aware of the newer and more likely nuclear disaster scenario – Nuclear Winter.

"In 1982, the so-called TTAPS team (Richard P. Turco, Owen Toon, Thomas P. Ackerman, James B. Pollack and Carl Sagan) undertook a computational modeling study of the atmospheric consequences of nuclear war, publishing their results in Science in December, 1983. The phrase "nuclear winter" was coined by Turco just prior to publication."[4]

Despite that -- the fact that nuclear winter might annihilate all human life and most edible vegetation -- my life went on. There was always hope.

Still, all through medical school and even in my first year of post-graduate internship, this concept of 'being useful even in times of disaster' tugged at me. My choice to become a primary care physician and then to specialize in OMM was actually based upon that specific criterion: What good would I be in the event of global disaster if I was isolated from hospitals and electricity and medicines? What could I learn that would make me more independent of the trappings of modern medicine and be truly USEFUL in a situation which would stymie most modern doctors who don't know how to make a diagnosis without their machines and technological tests and don't know how to treat someone for even the slightest problem, let alone serious illness or injury, without all of their modern equipment and medicines?

In the many years since Alas, Babylon and The Day After, we have been entertained by (or subjected to, depending upon your viewpoint) movies of local and wilderness and global disaster where people are left either individually, or in communities, to fend for themselves or to work together to survive. From one of my favorite global disaster movies with Dennis Quaid and Jake Gyllenhal, The Day After Tomorrow, to Steven King's

The Stand, to TV series like Lost, and yes, The Walking Dead – we have learned what brings out the best and the worst in people and are confronted with many choices and the ultimate question: Can we, as individuals and as a community, survive? Will we even choose to survive, if presented with a world gone mad with disease or war or natural disaster?

We may be confronted with such diverse challenges as weather changes, terrorist attacks, or solar ejection masses that will fry our electronics and with them, our way of modern life. If we do survive – will we be a taker, a boot-quaker, a leader, a soldier, a mechanic, inventor, builder, farmer, hunter, or … maybe even a healer?

It is with this in mind, that I present the case for osteopathic medicine in the context of disaster – local or global, Zombie or natural, and provide you with some insight into what osteopathic medicine is and why I believe it is what the modern world needs.

In addition to enjoying my disaster movies and series, I actually recently viewed a lecture by Dr. Abraham Verghese (http://www.ted.com/talks/lang/en/abraham_verghese_a_doctor_s_touch.html) about the human quality needed in medicine. Properly practiced, true osteopathy exemplifies this way of practicing – bonding with our patients in ways many of our colleagues in the allopathic community would consider 'crossing the line' or even misconduct. In disaster, a DO's job may not be just healing the body, but being part of the community, maybe even one of the bases for community and for civilized survival. Unlike Dr. Verghese, many doctors have simply forgotten their roots.

But we osteopaths – we TRUE osteopaths – we remember.

OVERVIEW OF WHAT WE'RE GOING TO COVER:

I. 20 of the Most Common Questions and Mis-Statements about Osteopathic Medicine.

In my 25 plus years of being an osteopathic physician, I have been asked many questions about my chosen profession; everything from, "You're a what??" to "Isn't a D.O an optometrist?" (That would be an O.D., Optometric Doctor) to "What is this manipulation stuff?"

The misinformation included statements such as, "Oh. You're a bone doctor," or "Ah, you're a chiropractor," "You're not a real doctor," and even, "That manipulation stuff is just quackery."

This section will simply list some of the most common questions and misconceptions. The answers will be found throughout the book.

II. The Basics of Osteopathic Medicine

This section will answer very basic questions about Osteopathic Medicine (Questions 1- 4, listed in the Section I: List of the TOP 20 QUESTIONS ABOUT OSTEOPATHIC MEDICINE) straight out, very briefly, to provide some background. Without this explanation, the scenarios that follow would likely make little sense.

III. Ground Rules of the Zombie Apocalypse:

Every disease has rules which it must follow. Every storyline also has rules.

I realize that many different stories and movies about Zombies have different rules from one another – are Zombies fast or slow? Can you get the disease by inhaling a virus from being near a zombie, being splattered by zombie blood or guts, or only if you are bitten? This section will lay out the ground rules of the disease of Zombism, as conceived for our purposes.

It is also unlikely that a Zombie Apocalypse will leave you in the vicinity of a working hospital with all the technology, testing facilities, conveniences, and the electricity to power them. As a result, this section will also designate what medical supplies are likely to be present and what tools you and your doctor(s) will have to work with to tend to your health needs and prevent you all from succumbing to the dreaded Zombie disease.

IV. Why You Should Care About Osteopathic Medicine:

In this section, the reader will be given scenarios that would likely occur in the event of a Zombie Apocalypse of global proportions. You will be faced with a series of challenges and will be asked to make choices, based upon what you know and believe. Each scenario will then be followed by the choices I believe best suit the situation along with an explanation of why each choice was made.

By the end of the book, the questions of 'Why you should care,' 'Why you might want to have an osteopathic physician with you at the end of all civilization,' or even simply, 'Why you should want an osteopathic physician to be your doctor – even if the world doesn't come to an end' - should be answered.

V. Why You Should Choose an Osteopathic Physician as Your Doctor, Especially as Your Primary Care Provider

VI. Why You Should Choose an Osteopathic Physician as Your Pain Specialist

VII. Little Known, but Very Cool Facts and Tidbits About Osteopathic Medicine

VIII. Helpful Resources

Where you can get more information on Osteopathic Medicine.

IX. Conclusion

X. Next Steps

What to do, now that you know all about Osteopathic Medicine.

Section I: List of the TOP 20 QUESTIONS ABOUT OSTEOPATHIC MEDICINE

1. Doesn't "Osteopath" just mean 'Bone Doctor'?
2. What, exactly, IS osteopathy?
3. What, exactly, is OMM?
4. What's the difference between an American Osteopathic Physician and a European Osteopath?
5. Is OMM only useful to treat pain?
6. How is OMM used to improve a patient's health?
7. Isn't osteopathy just quackery?
8. Is osteopathy and/or osteopathic medicine 'pseudoscience'?
9. What is the difference between chiropractic and osteopathic manipulation?
10. What's the difference between a D.O. and a D.C?
11. What's the difference between a D.O. and a physical therapist?
12. What's the difference between a D.O. and an M.D.?
13. How will osteopathic treatment differ from allopathic treatment?
14. What advantage(s) does osteopathic medicine offer over allopathic medical care?
15. Can OMM really help with non-musculoskeletal processes?
16. Should OMT be used as a first-line treatment or should it just be used as a tool to streamline diagnosis?
17. How would the various medical types treat disease and/or pain – acute and chronic?
18. Is OMM harmful in any way?
19. If osteopathic medicine is so wonderful, including OMT, why do so many osteopathic physicians NOT use it or use it only very little?
20. Why should I even care about osteopathic medicine if there's so much prejudice and misconception about it? In other words, What's In It For Me?

Section II: THE BASICS OF OSTEOPATHIC MEDICINE

1. Doesn't "Osteopath" just mean 'Bone Doctor'?

    Technically, yes. 'Osteo' is Greek for 'bone' and 'path' means 'disease or disorder.' Therefore, it sounds like osteopaths take care of bone diseases.

    What it actually means, though, is that osteopaths see the skeleton, as well as the muscles that move it, as a very important organ system. This 'musculoskeletal system' is, by mass, actually the largest organ system in the body. Moreover, all the other organs – from the skin, on the outside, to the brain, lungs, heart, and all the other organs on the inside – are encased within, hung from, supported by, moved, and fed by the musculoskeletal system.

    DO's also consider the nerves (which exit the spinal cord via openings between the vertebrae), as well as all the blood vessels of the body, to be vital. Even the lymphatic vessels (which are little-known, but crucial to the maintenance of fluid balance and immunity) travel through the narrow spaces between muscle sheets and within tight, confined spaces around bones, as well as within the connective tissue which I always liken to 'The Force' in Star Wars. This connective tissue (the white stuff in red meat and the stringy sheets seen when you lift the skin up off uncooked chicken parts) surrounds everything in the body, it penetrates all tissues, and binds us all together.

    The nerves and vessels are subject to all kinds of forces: stretching, twisting, and compression, which affect their functioning. Chiropractors, in theory, tend to focus on the nerves as they exit the spinal cord, believing that compression or twisting at the crucial point of exit is a major, if not the major, cause of abnormal nerve function. It is my understanding that this is why they emphasize 'spinal alignment' – to allow proper, free-flowing nerve impulses. It is, they feel, nerves which ultimately control all the major systems of the body. By improving nerve function, they improve everything from pain to immunity.

DO's, in theory, tend to harken back to osteopathy's founder, Andrew Taylor Still, who coined the saying, "The rule of the artery is supreme." Supposedly, osteopathic physicians are supposed to believe that it is blood flow which is more important in maintaining health and function of all parts and organ systems. Historically, DO's moved the spine, muscles, and bones to take the stresses off arteries and veins to improve blood flow. This maintained the flow of nutrients, oxygen, and immune cells to tissues, thereby improving health. As a consequence, improved blood flow to the nerves helped the nerves function properly.

In practice, today's modern osteopath and many of the best chiropractors I know, recognize that freeing both the nerves and blood vessels from strain, stress, stretching, impingement, or compression is necessary and vital to the achievement and maintenance of health and a well-functioning body.

2. What, exactly, is OMM?

    Most people are familiar with chiropractic manipulation. The most common forms I have experienced are the 'cracking' manipulation, usually of the spine, and use of 'activators' – small mechanical thumpers which help align spinal segments. There are other techniques used, by some, as well.

    OMM (Osteopathic Manipulative Medicine, also known as OMT, Osteopathic Manipulative Treatment or Therapy) is the application of specific forces, in very specific amounts and directions to tissues (bone, muscle, connective tissue, organs) to effect improved bodily function. Many DO's use chiropractic-style 'cracking' techniques. Many others use positioning techniques which require the patient to exert a force which the DO 'resists' in order to get the patient's own muscles to help re-align body parts. Many highly skilled DOs also use a large variety or other, more subtle and exceptionally effective techniques to help re-align parts of the body or allow the body to fix itself.

Allowing the body to fix itself is actually the ultimate goal of osteopathic medicine. If we can just help the body reduce its mechanical stresses and open the pathways for blood and lymph flow and decompress nerves so that they can function more fully, the body can usually heal itself much better and more fully than we can do by just introducing drugs into the system.

OMM is, therefore, a system of palpatory diagnosis (using our sense of touch to diagnose) and manual (hands-on) treatment.

The main difference between osteopathic manipulation and chiropractic is not so much the techniques used, but the focus of treatment.

I'm sure I'll get letters of correction from some very fine chiropractors, but I have had experience with enough DC's to know that the majority have the following foci:
    a.   Speed of treatment. With exceptions granted, the great majority of chiropractic treatments last under 10 minutes, most last under 5 minutes.
    b.   The spine is, for most, the only part of the body treated (again, exceptions granted).

c. Repeated treatment, often at specific time intervals, usually of the same area(s) of the spine, until the offending area is essentially trained to stay in place.

For DO's, the focus of treatment is: <u>completeness</u>.

Since DO's view the body and all its parts as an integrated unit, OMM seeks to treat all areas of the body where function or restriction are found, not just the spine. The idea is to improve flow of nutrients to, waste from, and neurological input to the affected areas to expedite self-healing.

At least some chiropractor's feel that DO's perform 'unnecessary' treatment. While chiropractors 'adjust' the spine, DO's 'treat' the whole body. We are taught to diagnose and treat dysfunction wherever we find it – from the bottoms of the feet to the top of the head and fingertip to fingertip, if necessary. We will even treat internal adhesions, which block flow or actually cause pain by directly pulling on pain-sensitive structures, when we can reasonably reach them.

Treating just the spine may work or it may not, though I have yet to figure out how it can loosen compressed connective tissue or break up adhesions which are pulling on pain-sensitive structures. Still, in the right hands, it may well work.

Removing impediments to blood, lymph, and neural flow throughout the body, however, and directly treating things like scars and adhesions, simply makes more sense to me. In fact, this aspect of osteopathic manipulation and the incredible mechanical logic behind it is what first drew me to osteopathic medicine and enticed me to research more about it. Ultimately, I have seen OMM work over and over again, throughout many, many years – even on disorders and pain which MD's and DC's were unable to help.

3. What are the <u>principles</u> of Osteopathic Medicine?

The American Osteopathic Association (the osteopathic counterpart to the AMA – American Medical Association – for MD's) says the following:

"Doctors of Osteopathic Medicine (DOs) are fully licensed physicians. They provide a full range of services, from <u>prescribing drugs to performing surgery</u>, and they <u>use the latest medical tools</u>. But DOs offer something special—their <u>unique approach to patient care</u>. Osteopathic physicians are trained to:

- teach patients how to **prevent illness and injury** by maintaining a healthy lifestyle.

- **look at the whole person** to reach a diagnosis without focusing just on symptoms.

- **help the body to heal itself**.

- believe that **all parts of the body work together** and influence one another. DOs are specially trained in the nervous system and the musculoskeletal system (muscles and bones).

- **perform** osteopathic manipulative treatment (OMT), a **hands-on** approach to **diagnosing, treating, and preventing illness or injury**."

Osteopathy also recognizes the body is an ***integrated unit of mind, body, and spirit***. Because of this, ideally, DO's take into account not just the person's physical well-being, but consider the less tangible aspects of emotional effects upon the body and the body's effects about the person's psychological well-

37

being. This is part of the 'whole body' or 'holistic' approach to people's healthcare which every DO is taught.

DO's are taught to **_LISTEN to our patients_** and their concerns. I can't tell you how many dozens or hundreds of times patients have complained to me about their MD's seeming too busy to listen to them or too disinterested in what they've had to say. DO's are taught this listening skill and as a result, learn a great deal more about empathizing with our patients. This empathy not only improves physician-patient relations, but actually contributes significantly to better patient care, in many ways, including improving the accuracy of our diagnoses.

4. What, exactly, IS osteopathy?

    and

5. What's the difference between an American Osteopathic Physician and a European Osteopath?

    I think this is a good place to make a distinction between 'osteopathy' and 'osteopathic medicine.'

    There is some difference of opinion between non-American osteopaths and American osteopathic physicians over just what 'osteopathy' is and what the founder of osteopathic medicine, Andrew Taylor Still, MD, meant it to be.

    Non-American osteopaths are generally not considered 'physicians' within their countries. They do not learn, or at least do not employ, all available diagnostic techniques, technologies, and treatments available to modern medicine. It is, I understand, their belief that Dr. Still intended osteopathy to be essentially only a manual diagnostic and treatment practice. They feel he meant to forgo all forms of pharmacological treatment, though I believe they accept some surgeries to be necessary.

As a result, however, two things are true about these non-American osteopaths:

  a. First, they choose not to utilize medication or surgery and are, therefore, legally barred from doing so within their countries.
  b. Since they only use manipulative medicine, but focus on the entire body as their manipulative domain, they are AMAZING at palpatory diagnosis and manipulative treatment. I have experienced their treatment and I will go as far as saying that their palpatory diagnostic and manipulative skills far surpass that of even some of the best-trained American osteopathic physicians. In fact, it is this recognition which inspired me to continually improve my manual medicine skills.

The American form of osteopathy, however, has evolved. American osteopathic medicine seeks to get rid of medications, but only those which don't work or which do more harm than good. Remember that at the inception of osteopathy, in the late 1800's, there was no FDA and no oversight regarding the safety of medications. Common treatments for ailments included such things as arsenic to treat infection. We American osteopaths are taught not to forgo all medications or all surgeries and technologies, but to choose and utilize the BEST of these diagnostic and treatment modalities – and to use them primarily when the body has lost the ability to heal itself, or perhaps needs some assistance to achieve self-healing.

All osteopaths are also taught that Dr. Still recognized that the body has within it, its own pharmacy, even though he did not know the specific chemicals such as antibodies, endorphins, endocannabinoids, etc. It was his recognition that manual treatment – removing the stresses and opening up the arterial pathways allowing these chemicals to flow – laid the basis for osteopathic manipulative therapy.

American 'osteopaths' however are true, full-fledged physicians and surgeons. As such, in order to learn all of what modern medicine has to offer, in addition to osteopathic manual diagnostics, principles, and practice, I'm afraid we do sacrifice the subtle and artistic skills which our foreign counterparts have. At the same time, though, we not only learn a great deal more – allowing us to write prescriptions and perform surgeries and opening up our eyes to all reasonable, available treatments – but, we may still avail ourselves of post-graduate study in manipulative medicine at outstanding residency and 'plus 1' post-graduate programs so that those interested can, in fact, master the more subtle manipulative diagnostic and treatment techniques'.

For those DO's already in practice who would still like to further their knowledge and skills in manual medicine, there are a number of wonderful continuing education courses to choose from. We may even choose to attend courses throughout the world which are taught by our non-American colleagues to pick up more of their excellent manual knowledge and skills.

As an American-trained osteopathic physician, when I utilize the term 'osteopath' or 'osteopathy' in this book, I am specifically referring to the American version of osteopathic medicine.

6. Is manipulation harmful? Can injuries occur from OMT?

The Truth: All treatments – medicine, surgery, even doing nothing (also known as 'watchful waiting' or 'expectant management') have risks associated with them. In choosing any treatment, the choice must be based on a benefit vs. risk analysis. In choosing a therapy, we always try to choose the one in which the benefits best outweigh the risks.

Surgery always carries a risk of infection, pneumonia, adverse reaction to anesthetic, and often death (even minor surgeries). Medications, even aspirin and acetaminophen (Tylenol™) have substantial risks including Reye's syndrome, kidney damage, and death. Consider the myriad attorney advertisements on late-night TV which recruit people injured by drugs. Both surgery and medicinal treatment generally carry a far greater risk than properly performed manipulation.

Yes, there have been complications associated with OMT or chiropractic, but many of these are preventable by using gentler types of manipulation. If properly done, OMT is generally considered exceptionally safe and very conservative. There are occasional injuries such as the rare lumbar disc herniation or stroke – but these are very few.*

The benefits of getting people moving, getting rid of their pain so they can run, shoot, turn their neck so they can see Zombies coming, fighting off infection, etc. far outweigh the potential risks of OMT.

---

* After researching many studies, I found the risks of severe injury from neck manipulation range from a very conservative 1 in 100,000[5] to 1 in 5.85 million[6]. Risk of worsening a lumbar disc herniation, even in a patient with pre-existing herniation of the disc, was found to be only 1 in 3.7 million[7]. And these are absolute worst-case scenarios. This is miniscule compared to the far more common serious risks associated with spinal surgeries including infection, hemorrhage and death. A recent study found life-threatening complications in older patients who underwent lumbar spinal fusion surgery may range between 2 and 3 PERCENT (1 in 33 to 1 in 50!)[8]

Section III: GROUND RULES OF THE ZOMBIE APOCALYPSE

1. We won't tackle preparedness for the Zombie Apocalypse in depth. We left that up to the United States Centers for Disease Control (CDC): http://www.cdc.gov/phpr/zombies.htm

2. Rather than giving you a list of supplies or ways to kill a zombie [you can always refer to The Zombie Survival Guide: Complete Protection from the Living Dead by Max Brooks] we'll focus on the medical aspects of Zombie Survival:
   a. Prevention of contracting Zombism and other diseases
   b. Treatment of early Zombie infections
   c. Other health issues you're likely to run into while on the run from your Zombie predators

3. About Zombism[9]
   a. All communicable illnesses take time to fully overcome their host's defenses
   b. Blood borne illnesses travel through the human body by catching a free ride on our fast-moving highway of arteries and veins
   c. For our purposes, the Rules Governing Zombism are:
      i. What is Zombism?
         a) Zombism is a bacterial infection which, after exposure and an incubation period, cause the patient to develop sepsis (wide-spread infection in the blood), pulmonary (lung) failure, and death ... followed by resurrection of a ravenous killing machine.
         b) The Zombie bacteria are resistant to all known antibiotics.

      ii. What does it take to become exposed?

a) A bite anywhere on the body is sufficient to cause infection.
b) You cannot get the disease by being splattered with bodily fluids or inhaling airborne particles.

iii. What is the incubation period?
The time from getting bitten to the first signs of infection is 2 days.

iv. What does the disease look like? What are the symptoms and the progression?
a) Within 2 days of being exposed to the bacteria, pulmonary (lung) symptoms begin and a fever develops.
b) At this time, the person becomes contagious, but only if he were to bite someone.
c) Within the next 24 hours, the person becomes nauseous, unable to take in fluids or food and severe muscle cramps develop.
d) The person becomes severely dehydrated and exchange of gases in the lungs becomes inhibited. Thick mucus plugs rapidly build in the lungs, further restricting airflow.
e) The time from getting the first pulmonary symptoms (shortness of breath, chest congestion) to complete dehydration, septic shock (too little fluid and a heavy bacterial toxin load causing the internal organs to shut down), pulmonary failure, and death is 3 days.
f) The time from death to resurrection is 6 hours.
g) Zombies do not think well and are attracted to smell, sound, and visual cues.
h) Zombies are quite steady on their feet and can walk quickly, but cannot run.
i) Contrary to the movies, Zombies don't have unending energy and are not particularly persistent. They want easy prey. They will work hard to capture and eat

someone/something for a few minutes, but beyond that, it uses too much energy and they will give up pursuit.

j) Also, contrary to the movies, even Zombies cannot live forever. As long as they can obtain meat (brains, for some) they will continue to survive to kill another day. If they go without eating for more than a month, however, they will eventually run out of energy and die.

v. What percentage of people exposed become infected?

a) As a general rule, not everyone exposed becomes infected. This is true of virtually all diseases. Some people may simply take more than one exposure to actually get the disease. Thus, some people have a certain level of resistance, but with sufficient exposure, everyone will eventually be overcome by the illness.

b) In this case, the bacteria are highly infective and 93% of people become ill after a single exposure. Experience has shown that those who survive the respiratory part of the illness do not go on to become Zombies. Very few, however, survive the respiratory illness since antibiotics are ineffective.

c) Finally, as is true with virtually all illnesses, a certain percentage of people will simply prove to be naturally immune to the infection or will develop the lung symptoms, but recover, becoming immune to the infection, though some could be considered carriers (if they bite someone ☺)

d) On the whole, however, 99+% of people who contract the illness become Zombies, hence the rapid spread of the illness.

4. Tools likely to be available in a disaster situation:

a. Being on the move to outrun Zombies, it is highly unlikely that survivors will have regular access to a fully stocked hospital or pharmacy.

b. Instead, survivors will likely have only whatever supplies they can scrounge from an urgent care facility, emergency room, or ambulance and can maintain only whatever they can carry with them either while on foot or in a vehicle, such as a van or ambulance.

c. With this in mind, we grant that survivors will have access to all of the following:

   i. basic IV equipment,

   ii. hydrating fluids like normal saline and dextrose

   iii. bandages

   iv. oxygen, tubing, and mask

   v. gauze

   vi. tape

   vii. tourniquets

   viii. a store of common antibiotics – cephalexin, amoxicillin/clavulanate (Augmentin™), trimethoprim/sulfamethoxazole (Bactrim™)

   ix. ibuprofen

   x. hydrocodone/acetaminophen (Vicodin™)

   xi. morphine

   xii. surgical supplies such as scalpel, sutures, and hemostats

   xiii. syringes and needles

   xiv. soap, antiseptics, iodine cleanser and non-iodine cleanser

   xv. Local anesthetic such as lidocaine vials

   xvi. Plaster

   xvii. ace wraps

   xviii. thermometer

   xix. blood pressure cuff

   xx. stethoscope

   xxi. tongue depressors

   xxii. Miscellaneous supplies such as forceps (tweezers), scissors, etc.

d. In addition, each type of doctor may have some supplies peculiar to them. An MD or DO may have an otoscope/ophthalmoscope for looking into people's eyes and ears. The DO may have some prolotherapy solution. A chiropractor may have an actuator.

5. How I chose what each professional is likely to use:
   a. based upon what the average student of that profession is taught through schooling and post-graduate professional training.
   b. based upon my personal experiences with each of the professions, having worked with and been treated by members of each of these professions.

Section IV: WHY YOU SHOULD CARE ABOUT OSTEOPATHIC MEDICINE:

As stated earlier, in this section, the reader will be given scenarios that would likely occur in the event of a Zombie Apocalypse of global proportions. I am going to ask you to look at each event **as if YOU WERE THE DOCTOR**. This will help you understand what the doctor sees, how he thinks, what challenges he faces when caring for patients like yourself, and, ultimately, **what kind of doctor YOU would want caring for YOU**, should a similar situation arise.

You will be faced with a series of challenges and will be asked to make choices, based upon what you know and believe. There is not always just one correct answer, so select all answers which you believe are likely to be correct. Each scenario will then be followed by the choices I believe best suit the situation along with an explanation of why each choice was made.

Some of the scenarios will, additionally, be followed with a real-life anecdote, usually from my personal experience, so that the reader can understand these are not wild-eyed, exaggerated stories which could never happen. In one form or another, they actually happen every day.

SCENARIO 1

The Zombie Apocalypse is fully under way. You are in a group of 20 people who are trapped in a bookstore at the edge of town. Outside, the streets are crawling with Zombies, but they are not concentrated in any one place. As a group, you decide that a mad dash of three blocks will take you to the edge of the city. Beyond that, you will be able to run through the forest and lose the Zombie horde among the trees. You figure that within a half mile, you will be free of the immediate Zombie threat.

Unfortunately, one of your number, an otherwise healthy looking woman in her early forties refuses to make the run. For the past 2 days she has had severe chest pain. Her doctors had not found a reason for it, but were concerned that she might have an as yet undetected problem with her heart. Others were worried that she might have been infected. (Her doctors are now dead, Zombified, or otherwise inaccessible.) She has been warned against excessive exertion. She fears that if she tries to outrun the Zombies, she may have a heart attack. It is difficult for her to breathe deeply, even at rest.

You are faced with the choice of everyone being stuck in your hideout until food and water run out or leaving her to fend for herself while you all make the mad dash to the woods. Of course, a few of you vote for throwing her, screaming, into the street as bait while the rest of you head for the trees.

You are the doctor in the group. You absolutely refuse to leave this woman behind or use her as bait. You foolishly believe that all human life is precious – and more practically, you never know what important contribution a member of the group might make at a crucial moment later along your survival trek. Besides, you might need her to help repopulate the human race once the Zombie scourge dies off, if it ever does.

CHOICES:

As the 'Doctor,' you have several determinations you can make. They are:

1. What kind of doctor are you?
   a. Chiropractor
   b. Dentist
   c. DO (Doctor of Osteopathic Medicine)
   d. MD

   Your Choice: _____

***

This is your short-list for differential diagnosis for the woman's condition? ('Differential Diagnosis' is 'doctor jargon' for 'what are the possible causes of her pain/condition?')
   a. Ischemic heart disease (i.e. she has 'angina' – chest pain which indicates she could have a heart attack at any moment)
   b. Early Zombism – pulmonary phase
   c. Dysfunctional Rib
   d. Asthma
   e. Psychologically induced pain
   f. Influenza
   g. Pneumonia

2. What procedure(s) test(s) might you use, which you have at your disposal, to determine what the woman's problem is?
   a. Tapping on her chest
   b. Listening to her lungs with a stethoscope while she sings "EEEEE"
   c. Asking her questions such as, "Have you been bitten recently by a Zombie?" or "Have you been around anyone with coughing or chest congestion, lately?"

d. Asking her "Does it hurt when you breathe in deeply and/or when you completely exhale?"
e. Measuring her temperature
f. Palpating (examining by touch) her chest wall
g. Put your palm on her face and say, "My mind to your mind…"

Your Choice(s): _____
[Answer on the next page:]

A through F are all correct.

a. Tapping on her chest

Tapping on a person's chest is called 'percussion'. An air-filled lung, when percussed, sounds like a hollow drum. If the person has pneumonia or pleurisy (fluid around the lung) the percussion produces a higher pitch at the site of the problem.

b. Listening to her lungs with a stethoscope while she sings "EEEEEE"

I bet this one surprised some of you. When a person has pneumonia or the lung is filled (consolidated) with fluids, mucus, or bacteria, the sound "EEEE" changes to the sound "AAAAA" (as in 'gate'). This is called egophany.

c. Asking her questions such as, "Have you been bitten recently by a Zombie?" or "Have you been around anyone with coughing or chest congestion, lately?"

I think this is common sense. If she wasn't bitten and you see no signs that she was, she is unlikely to be infected with the Zombie bacteria, sparing you the necessity of killing her or throwing her out as bait. She could, however, have the flu or other respiratory illness.

d. Asking her "Does it hurt when you breathe in deeply and/or when you completely exhale?"

This is a somewhat tricky question. You want to know not only if it hurts when she breathes in or out, but where it hurts. Does it hurt deep inside her chest (chest congestion) or does it hurt only in the wall of her chest in the front and/or in her back? Pain only in the chest wall is a clue that the pain may not be in the lung or heart, at all, but in the muscles or skeleton of the chest. You'll also want to know if the pain goes away when she rests. If it does, then it may only be hurting when her heart is under stress, indicating possible heart disease. If it doesn't go away with rest, the pain is likely to be caused by something other than heart disease.

e. Measuring her temperature

Without fever, there is a greater likelihood that the problem is not infectious. Palpating (examining by touch) her chest wall.

f. Palpating (examining by touch) her chest wall

I can't tell you how many times a patient came into the emergency room with chest pain and the doctors I was working under never touched them. After one look at the patient, a panel of blood tests, EKGs, and even x-rays would be ordered. These are fine precautions in an ER, but I also can't tell you how many times I put my hands on a person's chest to see if I could reproduce the pain or to see whether I could feel whether or not a rib was stuck. 9 times out of 10, if I could simply reproduce the pain with my hands, the person had chest wall pain coming from the rib cage and not heart problems.

What each type of doctor is likely to do:

MD:

Here's a clue: most MD's I've known won't even do 'a' through 'e' under normal circumstances and only one I have ever come across would even attempt 'f' – and that's only because he had been trained by osteopaths.

DC (chiropractor):

Chiropractors might do 'a' through 'f' as well – but only very well-trained DC's.

By the way, 'g' for those of you who don't know, is how a Vulcan mind-meld is initiated.

DO:

A well-trained and properly practicing osteopathic doctor would do all of these tests, if necessary (excluding the mind-meld).

[Next page:]

Having done your tests, because you're an amazing doctor, you have found the following:

> Percussion is normal. She has no egophany and her lungs sound clear under the stethoscope. She has no fever. She has not been around anyone with the flu and has not been bitten by a Zombie. Her pain does not go away with rest. In fact, it never really changes. Palpation reproduces her pain and you find that she has a rib which is 'stuck' in expiration, meaning that every time she inhales, that rib doesn't move and it causes her pain.
>
> Diagnosis: Dysfunctional rib.

3. Now that you know what the problem is, how do you treat it?
    a. Give her Vicodin™ or Ibuprofen and wait for the medicine to work before you all dash to the woods.
    b. Fix her spine.
    c. Fix the rib so that it moves, again, and then head for the woods.
    d. Throw her into the street as Zombie bait and head for the woods.

Your Choice(s): _____

[Next Page]

DC:

Fix her spine and hope that fixes her pain, although I have known some excellent chiropractors who are well-versed in fixing ribs, as well.

MD:

You give her the Vicodin™ and/or Ibuprofen, depleting what small stores you have of the medications – which you might need for more serious problems in the future – and hope it eases the pain. Sometimes it works, sometimes it doesn't. In the end, however, her pain will return full force within a few hours and you'll need to dose her, again, every time you want to run – except you might not get as much time to prepare to run as you have at this moment, in which case, she's looking much more like Zombie-bait.

DO:

You definitely fix both the spine, if affected, and the rib cage (at least). If that completely relieves her pain, you're done and everybody starts running. If it relieves some of her pain, you may choose to dose her with medication so you can all leave within the hour when it takes effect. If the pain comes back, however, once you're all safe and have more time, you can do a more thorough examination, including a full-body musculoskeletal exam. At that point, you can treat all the restrictions you find that could be contributing to her chest wall pain, pulling on the rib or muscles, and preventing that rib from functioning. Once fixed, she'll be ready to run on a moment's notice the next time a trot becomes necessary.

Real-life:

The following is a true story:

One day, as I was walking up the steps to my dentist's office, I received a call. Without exaggeration, the woman on the line sounded desperate. This is what she told me:

"Doctor, I've had pain in my chest for nearly four months. I've had every test known to man and still the doctors have found nothing. I've been to my own doctor, the lung doctor, and the cardiologist. The pain is horrible. I'm at my wits' end. Today they took blood to run nearly a hundred tests. If they don't find anything, I don't know what I'll do.

I came across your ad in the yellow pages as someone who deals with pain. You're my last hope."

To be honest, I seemed to be everybody's last hope because they went to all the 'real' doctors, first. When the 'real' doctors couldn't help them, they finally turned to me.

I said, "Ma'am. Can I ask you a couple of questions? Is the pain sharp, burning, dull, or pressure-like?"

"Sharp," she said. "Very sharp."

"Does it ever go away? When you rest, for instance?"

"Not really. No."

I had an idea what was going on. "I see," I continued. "Does it hurt in front or in back or both?"

"Both," she answered.

"Mmm hmm. And does it hurt when you take a deep breath all the way in?"

"Oh, YES!" she exclaimed. "Terrible, just terrible."

"Does it hurt when you exhale all the way?"

"Oh, YES!"

"Ma'am," I said, "I suspect you have a rib out of whack. Why don't you come in at 2:30 tomorrow afternoon and I'll see what we can do. If I'm wrong, you've lost nothing. If I'm right, your pain should resolve quickly."

"Oh, THANK YOU!" she said. "I'll be there."

I went into the office pretty pleased with myself.

The next morning, however, at 9:00 AM, I got a call. It was the woman with chest pain. "Doctor, I'm afraid I'll have to cancel our appointment, today."

"Oh?" I asked, "Why?"

(I'm actually quoting her, here.) "Well, she said, "Those blood tests came back and one of them was slightly off. I want to go to the cardiologist before we go any further."

"I see," I said. "Before you decide, I'd like to point out two things, though. First, nobody's blood tests are perfect all the time. At any given moment, there will be slight variations and slight deviations from normal. If you take a hundred blood tests, it is likely that at least one or two at any given minute will fall slightly outside the 'normal' range.

Second, you can still see the cardiologist, but it makes sense to come in for diagnosis and possible treatment. It's all non-invasive and won't hurt you. If we fix it, your troubles are over. If we don't, you can still continue with the cardiologist and have all the tests or treatments he recommends."

What did she say??

"No. No. I'm going to see the cardiologist. Thank you, anyway."

I never did see that lady.

But, that's not the end of the story. There is a more interesting moral.

I went home, saddened but bemused. I have four children. At the time, my oldest was about 16 and my youngest was 7. I told them each the story, individually, without telling them what I thought was going on and asked them what they thought.

When I told my daughter, the oldest, she said, "She's got a rib out of place." I smiled.

Throughout the evening, I went down the line and asked each of my three boys what they thought about the story. Right down to my 7 year old, they each said, "She's got a rib out of whack."

This is the moral: Why couldn't this woman's doctors make that diagnosis when even a child could do it?

Her doctors needed to know about body-mechanics and needed to know the diagnosis of 'rib dysfunction' even existed before they could consider it in their differential diagnosis. My kids, however, grew up with an osteopath for a father and were well aware that the diagnosis existed.

The moral: What your MD doesn't know can hurt you.

From the movie, "Alien Apocalypse", written and directed by Josh Becker and starring Bruce Campbell as Dr. Ivan Hood, D.O.* [10]

[After 40 years in suspended animation in space, Dr. Ivan Hood and his team return to an Earth taken over and decimated by insect-like aliens. The few remaining humans are either slaves or live free in primitive conditions reminiscent of the dark ages.]

IVAN
[very drunk]
. . . Ever since I was a kid I wanted to be a doctor. I'd watch "E.R." and "Marcus Welby" reruns on TV and think, "I wanna be like that . . . "

ALEX
What's TV?

IVAN
None of your business.

But my grades weren't good enough, so I joined the Air Force, figured I'd fly jets, or helicopters, or something . . . But no . . . My grades weren't good enough for that, either. Luckily, they put me through Osteopathic school, but all the M.D.s treated D.O.s like they were quacks. And then I ended up on that stupid space mission 'cause no "real" doctors wanted to go away for [forty] years. I figured I'd come back to a better world a hero, but no . . .

[Ivan sighs deeply, drops over backward and passes out.]

----

*It should be noted that although Dr. Hood is a caricature of an osteopathic physician, which makes him funny and appealing as a movie character, many of the things he does and says represent, in a seriocomic fashion, many of the daily struggles DO's actually face.

SCENARIO 2

You've all made it safely to the woods. The lady's chest pain is resolved and she led the pack high-tailing it out of town.

As you take a moment to rest, though, a young man, maybe 30 years old seems to be gasping for air. He knows he has asthma. His doctors diagnosed it. He uses his steroid inhaler as scheduled and his lungs were nearly clear (just a little wheezy) before the dash. Now that he's run so far, he's wheezing very heavily and reaches into his backpack for his rescue-inhaler. He takes a few puffs and within minutes, he's breathing easier, though he still feels like he's wheezing a little.

"I'll be all right," he says, bravely. "I'm always a little wheezy."

"Really?" you ask, with grave concern. "How many of those inhalers do you have with you?"

"Just one steroid inhaler and one rescue inhaler, for the times when the wheezing gets really bad," he answers.

"How long will that all last you," you ask.

"The steroid inhaler will last about another week. I'll run out of the rescue medicine well before that," he replies.

You're the doctor. I know you're concerned. Without his medications, he'll most likely die within the next week.

Now, I also know you've become a good listener – you listened to the first lady with the chest pain and figured out how to help her, right? How can you help this young man? CAN you help him?

CHOICES:
1.   Again, what kind of doctor will you choose to be?
     a. Chiropractor
     b. Dentist
     c. DO
     d. MD

Your Choice: _____

2.   What can you do to figure out if you can help this young man and keep him alive when his medicines run out?

[NEXT PAGE]

MD:

Prayer.

You're not really interested in his history because you know the history is irrelevant for 3 reasons:
1. Asthma can't be brought on by trauma or other physical problems. It's just not possible. People with asthma generally have some kind of genetic defect which causes their airways to over-react to stimuli such as allergens (like pollen or dust) or even weather changes.
2. The only way to properly treat asthma is with appropriate medications.
3. If it were brought on by trauma or some other physical stimulus (by some fluke), you wouldn't know how to fix it, anyway.

DC:

Take a history. You understand that trauma CAN cause asthma-like symptoms. Maybe there will be a clue as to the cause of the symptoms.

DO:

You DEFINITELY start with a thorough history! It is drilled into every DO's head that 85% of all diagnoses can be made from a thorough history. You will be looking not only for traumatic problems, but also emotional problems which can trigger asthma-like symptoms - called somatoform disorders (as if running from Zombies and the end of civilization weren't sufficient emotional traumas!) and any other clues which might lead you to a treatable condition. This man's life is in your hands!

As you sit on a boulder and he paces to keep his chest erect and his airways maximally open, you ask him some questions and listen carefully to the answers.

"Tell me about your asthma. When did it start?"

"It started about 3 years ago," he replies.

"Only 3 years ago??" you ask, incredulous. "Usually, if you're going to get asthma as a young person, it doesn't start in your 20's. It's usually first seen when you're much younger."

"Yeah, I know," he says. "It's the weirdest thing. The doctors were kind of puzzled, too."

"Do you have allergies?" you ask. "Allergies, even in older people, can sometimes trigger asthma or asthma-like symptoms."

"Nope. Never had allergies. The docs tested me for that," he says.

Curious, you feel the need to probe. "Tell me about how it started. What was it like?"

"Well, that's the weird thing. I was healthy as a horse all my life. Three years ago, I was out riding my motorcycle when I was hit by a car. I was thrown from the bike but it was a miracle! I actually landed on my feet! Both my feet were badly broken, but the rest of me hadn't a scratch. It was amazing. I was real lucky.

The funny thing is, about two or three months later, I started having breathing problems. I took a bunch of tests and they measured my lung function. They weren't sure, but thought it looked like asthma. I've been wheezing ever since."

Now, you know this fellow hasn't long to live without your help. What can you do for him? Ok, Doctor, what are you thinking? What's your next step?

    a.   Hope someone has some marijuana with them
    b.   Find turmeric seasoning as soon as possible
    c.   Pray
    d.   Determine how tasty the Zombies will find his dead carcass

Your Choice(s): _____

[NEXT PAGE]

MD:

Well, if you're an MD, there's not much you can do. The only thing you know how to do for his condition is to prescribe medicines.

Hey, WAIT A MINUTE! You remember you brought along a book you grabbed from the bookstore; it's all about edible and medicinal plants.[‡] (Good Job! – not that you normally ascribe to the use of such natural treatments, but ... hey, desperate times require desperate measures!)

Maybe, depending upon the season and your locale, you might be able to scrounge up some appropriate plants and brew up a concoction that will sustain this guy, at least until winter comes. Of course, none of these treatments are as potent as steroids or the medicines in rescue inhalers, but it's something.

DC:

If you're a chiropractor – and you're not one reliant on x-rays to make your diagnoses – you might be able to find and fix problems in his spine as well as his ribs or pelvis if they're out of whack.

In fact, knowing the history, you might suspect that the impact really jarred things and perhaps that impact set his spinal segments askew, causing asthma-like symptoms. You could well be correct or at least not far off the mark.

In addition, there would be no reason you could not utilize the available plant-life if you have the book or prior knowledge of medicinal plants.

DO:

As a DO, you could utilize medicinal plant knowledge, since you have the book. You grabbed it, of course, not just out of desperation, but because you have been taught that most medications have their roots in botanicals. You knew that information would eventually come in handy, so you never hesitated to consider the book a great resource.

You already know that if you can get hold of some turmeric (an herbal seasoning) maybe from a house's spice rack, if you come across one, it's been used by inhabitants of India to help with asthma for centuries.

If you're well-rounded and haven't been blinded by the lies of Big Pharma and can make intelligent, evidence-based decisions for yourself, you also know that marijuana is actually a good choice. Its muscle relaxant and anti-inflammatory properties make it quite suitable as a treatment for asthma.

The problem is that even if your herbal remedies would work, first you have to have some with you or you'd better find some, fast. Eventually, though, you run the risk of running out of the herbal medications quite quickly.

Having heard the history, you are considering other causes for this young man's late-blooming asthma. You decide to do a thorough physical examination – another vital task of EVERY MEDICAL ENCOUNTER – as has been drummed into your osteopathic head since the first day you entered medical school.

As a DO, you realize that trauma could, in fact, cause asthma-like symptoms. A physical examination could be very revealing. You can treat any spinal problems you find – and most definitely any rib restrictions or pelvic problems you find. But, as a DO, you might also realize that restrictions in the chest can be caused by tissues twisting or malfunctioning almost anywhere in the body – including in the feet (which, in this case, have been severely traumatized).

Remember how the fascia – the connective tissue of the body – is like 'the Force' in Star Wars? It surrounds us, penetrates us, and binds us all together. Every muscle, every bone, every organ is surrounded, penetrated and bounded by this connective tissue.

Another analogy I use for this fascia is plastic wrap (like Saran Wrap™). Think of a big sheet of plastic wrap, laid out on the floor. If you twist a corner of the plastic, you will see ripple emanating from that point all the way out to most of the sheet. The same thing happens in the body; a restriction in some distant part of the body, such as the lower extremity or pelvis, might put torque and stress on tissues – far away from the source of actual injury.

In order to successfully straighten out the whole sheet (or body), however, it would require you to not only straighten out the far edges, but you would have to go back to the point where the ripples originate and straighten that out, as well.

A good osteopath can find the source of the ripples.

You decide to do a thorough examination of this gentleman and find not only the problems in his upper body – spine and ribs – but you also find problems in his pelvis and lower extremities. It seems the right half of the pelvis has shifted upward relative to the left half. You theorize this was due to the impact, three years ago. If you are successful at repositioning the pelvic halves and straightening out any spinal, rib, and lower extremity problems which resulted from the trauma, this man might just survive the loss of his medications.

REAL LIFE:

Story 1:
Well, this REALLY HAPPENED to a friend of mine. He was actually the passenger on a motorcycle when the bike was hit. He landed on his feet which were badly broken. A few months later, he was diagnosed with asthma. He and I met three years after his accident.

Unlike our young man in this story, however, his asthma wasn't mild. It became severe enough to require him to be on chronic oral steroids (prednisone) as well as maintenance and rescue inhalers. Steroids, if you're not aware, are very useful medications. Unfortunately, they also have a number of really bad side-effects from causing mood-swings, to inhibiting your immune system, to causing severe weight-gain, making your skin thin and fragile, and even, ultimately, damaging your lungs (which was, in this case, what they were supposed to be protecting!).

In my friend's case, I was able to diagnose the problem and fix it. Within a month, he was off ALL steroids and all asthma medications. His MD's were frankly astounded and didn't hesitate to let him know.

Until we finally lost touch, whenever he would begin to wheeze a little bit, he would call me right away so that I could perform OMT and fix the problem.

Ideally, of course, it would have been nice to stop the problem from ever recurring. I could have done that, but we never got the chance. How we could have done that, however, is a story for another time.

‡I'm from Michigan, so a great book might be <u>Edible and Medicinal Plants of the Great Lakes Region</u>, by Thomas A. Naegele, D.O.

Story 2:

The second point that needs to be made is that as an osteopathic doctor, you should be concerned with more than just the patient's historical and physical findings. Emotional triggers and crises of spirit or conscience can have a significant effect on the patient's health. In the above scenario, you are advised to be looking for such triggers. Here's why:

About 30 years ago, a 40-something year-old woman was escorted to the doctor's office by her 21 year old son. She'd been having chest pains for a few days. She thought maybe she was having heart problems.

Upon arriving at the doctor's office, the doctor took a careful history and did an appropriate physical examination. The EKG was ok. Her lungs were clear and he could find no physical problem. He sat down and talked to her and said, "Tell me what's really bothering you."

She looked at her son and asked him to leave. The doctor caught the look and said, "No. Stay." He then asked again, "Tell me what's really bothering you."

Over the next 10 minutes this woman cried and poured out her concerns over choices her son was making. She was concerned about his schooling and his future. The son and his mother then talked things through with the doctor mediating the discussion. Miraculously, her chest pain resolved.

Psychological, social, emotional, and spiritual factors can have an immense impact on someone's health. Contrary to popular belief, that doesn't make a person 'crazy.' The health problems or pain caused by the emotional triggers is quite real.

The stress reaction triggers pain sensors to fire, triggers nerves which control blood pressure and muscle tension to fire. It triggers the release of cortisol from the adrenal gland which affects mood, sense of well-being, blood sugar levels, and immune function, pre-disposing people to bouts of shingles, cold sores, infections, and yes, heart disturbances. Lung function can be affected, simulating asthmatic symptoms; and so much more.

It is vital that such stressors be considered by a good physician. DO's are always taught to make these considerations.

By the way, Mom is fine.

And so am I.

SCENARIO 3

You little group has survived mostly by pilfering what you could from available vehicles or homes, by eating edible plants which you've identified with the help of your Edible and Medicinal Plants book, and because one member of your group has always been an active outdoorsman ... er, outdoorsperson. It turns out that the lady you saved from being a Zombie sandwich back at the bookstore has proven vital to your survival. She is your tracker and hunter. She has been hunting and trapping small game along the way. As long as she does her job, food is fairly plentiful, though many of you have been grossed out by the skinning chores and the smell of raw intestinal contents from the game.

Your hunter-tracker is trailing a deer, today, which could feed the small community for a week, after drying and curing the meat. The bones could also be made into everything from tools to fertilizer (for future use). Unfortunately, she stumbles down a small ravine, twists her ankle and injures her knee. She also receives a big gash in her thigh which partially severs her quadriceps muscle and which is exposed to dirt. If she's out of action for long, you may all go hungry or even starve. In the meantime, you need to keep moving.

Choose your profession:
- a. Chiropractor
- b. Dentist
- c. DO
- d. MD

Your Choice: _____

The injuries are pretty obvious, so there are no great diagnostic dilemmas, here. The problem is one of urgency: She can't be out of commission for very long or you're all going to get pretty protein-deficient. More importantly, that open wound presents a problem: it's dirty and is almost certain to become infected if not cared for, immediately.

What will you do?

DC:

As a chiropractor, you can assess it the injuries. Depending upon your education and experience – and how much first-aid you know – you may be able clean the wound out with soap and water and/or lots of sterile saline (you have it with you). You may be able to manipulate the ankle and knee to realign the bones, to make them more functional and heal more quickly, or you may not.

Can you sew the muscle belly together? Can you close the subcutaneous fat and then the skin? Do you WANT to? (Sometimes, it's better to leave a dirty wound open and let it close itself, naturally. As a chiropractor, are you trained to know this?

If you decide to give prophylactic antibiotics (to prevent infection) do you know which antibiotic(s) to choose from your stock and the dosages to use?

MD:

You can assess whether the knee and ankle are broken or whether a ligament is partially or completely torn. You can splint the joints, if you think it's necessary. You can certainly clean the wound and probably sew the partially severed muscle back together. You most likely will be able to rationally decide whether to close the wound or to let it heal by secondary intention (meaning let it heal and close on its own, without sewing it closed). You will most likely be able to determine which, if any, antibiotics to use and what dosages.

Unfortunately, nothing you do will actually help get the huntress back in the field particularly quickly. In fact, the constant pain might even slow your entire party down.

Both you and the chiropractor (if he's progressive) might recommend NSAIDS (non-steroidal anti-inflammatory agents) such as ibuprofen for the pain, as well. In addition, you might use the opiates (narcotics) you have available to help with the pain.

DO:

Well, a DO can do everything the chiropractor can do – and so much more. As a DO, you can also do what the MD can do … and quite a bit more.

Specifically, in addition to all of the above, a DO can reset the talus in the mortis (reset the ankle), but it is commonly taught to DO's that the fibular head (up by the knee) must be checked and reset whenever the ankle is sprained, because spraining the ankle tends to pull the fibular head away from its normal position at the knee. This malpositioning may well prevent the ankle from improving and substantially lengthen the healing time. Treating both the ankle injury, itself, and the fibula could help get the huntress up and working, again, significantly more quickly than if only the ankle were treated.

In addition, you would manipulate the limb (as tolerated) as well as other vital areas of the body to improve the immune function to help it fight off infection and to improve blood flow to and from the affected areas (to increase nutrient flow into the area and removal of waste products from the area) to decrease healing time..

One final difference between MD's and DO's might be the withholding of anti-inflammatory medications. Not all DO's agree, but many do (as do some MD's). The body actually heals through the process of inflammation. Taking NSAIDS can interfere with that healing process. As a result, you might prefer just to use the Vicodin™ or morphine to control pain.

All of this gives your huntress the best chance at the fastest and smoothest recovery.

REAL LIFE:

My son was playing baseball. He was the first baseman. While catching the ball thrown to him, the runner bowled into him, injuring my son's knee. The ligament on the inside of his knee was partially torn, but not severely. Still, he was in a great deal of pain and couldn't move his knee. Usually, this kind of injury can take 3 weeks or more to improve enough to allow a player back into the game.

Immediately, I went over to him and had him grit his teeth as I reset the bones in his knee and checked the bones in his ankle, as well. He had instantaneous relief of most of the pain, but I took him out of the game for a week. Since I withheld NSAIDS from him, (NSAIDS impede ligament healing) he was able to return to play within a week.

Another example: I, myself, experienced a disc herniation in my lower back. I have never had such intense pain. I could not stand or sit. I spent most of my time standing behind a couch, bent over the back of the couch. This was the only position which relieved the pain, at all. It sounds crazy, I know, but that's the truth.

Now, here is the interesting part:

Standard treatment for herniated discs includes the administration of NSAIDS and narcotic pain relievers. To relieve extreme pain, sometimes steroids are used, as well.

Unfortunately, the NSAIDS, while reducing the pain immensely, interfere with the body's ability to heal itself. Steroids interfere with the healing process even more than the NSAIDS. As a result, most people who take the NSAIDS have a significantly prolonged healing time for their disc injuries, on the order of 6-12 weeks. Moreover, healing is frequently left incomplete because of the interference of the NSAIDS. Consequently, the patients are left with residual, sometimes life-long, pain.

Another standard approach, unfortunately, is to perform a surgery called a laminectomy to relieve the pain and pressure on nerves exiting the spinal cord. The consequences of this can be disastrous with scarring and even more pain and disability than before the surgery. Again, the consequences can be life-long.

Personally, I chose to live on narcotic pain killers for 3 weeks and avoid all NSAIDs. BUT, after 3 weeks, my pain had completely disappeared, I was completely healed, and I have never had any residual problems from that once-herniated disc.

BAKER
This fella here [indicating IVAN] says he's a spaceman.

(A big man with strong arms and reddish hair stands up rather crookedly. He is ISAAC. Ivan steps up to him.)

IVAN
Second Lieutenant Ivan Hood, D.O.
Who're you?

ISAAC
I am Isaac. I am the leader of Freedom Valley.

IVAN
Nice to meet you...

ISAAC
What does D.O. mean?

IVAN
I'm a Doctor of Osteopathy.

ISAAC
Does that mean you are a doctor for animals or humans?

IVAN
(sarcastically)
Osteopathy is the study of slugs and their mating habits.

ISAAC
(eyes light up)
Really? I've always been interested in slugs. How do they mate?

IVAN
Very carefully.

SCENARIO 4

A young woman in your group who has mostly kept to herself since the start of your journey woke up this morning with complaints of severe abdominal pain. She didn't want to complain, at first, but finally, she sought you out.

"How long have you had the pain?" you ask.

"Just since this morning, sir." (Sir??)

"Are you nauseous?"

"Yes, sir. Very," she says.

"Where is the pain, exactly?" you inquire.

She puts her hand over the center of her abdomen, "Here."

"May I?"

She nods.

Choose your profession:
   a. Chiropractor
   b. Dentist
   c. DO
   d. MD

   Your Choice: _____

You put on the stethoscope and listen to her abdomen (Dentist or maybe chiropractor). You know that normally, the tummy is always gurgling at least a little bit. When you hear no gurgling in her abdomen, at all, you begin to get concerned.

Here are some possible diagnoses:
   1. Appendicitis
   2. Viral enteritis (intestinal infection)
   3. Pancreatitis
   4. Food poisoning
   5. Severe Constipation
   6. Strep throat (causes fever, chills, sore throat, and
      severe abdominal pain)

What do you do, next?

[NEXT PAGE]

You might start by getting a bit more history (you should know this, by now!)

This is the information you get:

She had a normal bowel movement yesterday. [Eliminates severe constipation as a probable cause.] She doesn't have pain anywhere else. She doesn't have a sore throat or any respiratory symptoms. [Rules out strep throat as a probable cause.] She hasn't had any chills. The onset was fairly sudden. She hasn't had any diarrhea or heartburn. [Makes food poisoning and intestinal infection less likely, but doesn't completely eliminate them as culprits.] She last ate more than 12 hours ago.

What do you do, next?

[NEXT PAGE]

DC:
> If you're a chiropractor – I honestly have no idea what you do next. Perhaps you want her to try an herbal medication and stay hydrated. Perhaps you provide a trial of chiropractic manipulation to see whether or not the intestines will begin to function again.

Unfortunately, she will not drink – she can't tolerate it. You ask, "If I offered you your favorite food in the whole world, right now, would you eat it?"

> She replies, "My favorite food in the world is pizza," (that went the way of the Dodo Bird with the current Zombie problem), "But even if you offered it to me, there's no way I could eat it."

> MD or DO:
>> You decide you need to do a more thorough physical exam. These are your findings:
>>
>> Most of her exam is normal. She has no swollen lymph nodes, including behind the ears or in the neck and her throat looks completely pink and healthy. [Rules out strep throat.] She does have a slight fever or 100.4° F. When you push on her abdomen, there are no enlarged organs and no pain or tenderness just below the breastbone. [This makes pancreatitis less likely.] When you push on her mid abdomen, there is no pain, but when you let go quickly, her pain is severe.

> What do you think is the cause, now?
>> Viral enteritis?
>> Appendicitis?

You can't do any lab tests, so you can't definitively rule in or rule out pancreatitis or determine whether she has a viral or bacterial infection.

A viral infection will most likely resolve on its own within a few days. Pancreatitis can be treated conservatively if you can just keep the patient hydrated and nourished, even if it's only with IV fluids. A bacterial infection or appendicitis (which is basically a bacterial infection of the appendix) can be very dangerous if not properly and promptly treated. If the intestine develops a hole in it (perforation) or an infected appendix bursts, the young woman will probably die of a massive infection of the abdomen (peritonitis).

What's your next step?

[NEXT PAGE]

You decide to wait.

WHAT?

She could die and we're just going to WAIT?

Yes, wait.

You can't take any tests and you can't just do an exploratory surgery. It's only been 12 hours since your patient last ate, so she won't likely starve to death. You need to watch her hydration. If she starts becoming too dehydrated, you can start an IV for fluids.

Her fever is not particularly high, yet, and her examination is fairly non-specific; i.e. it doesn't tell you much. You don't even know whether antibiotics are warranted (and you need to conserve your supply, if you can) because if it's a viral enteritis, it will resolve on its own and antibiotics don't work on viruses. Also, antibiotics aren't generally effective against appendicitis.

In this case, waiting and watching may be the best course of action.

***

About 6 hours later, her pain has increased and her temperature has gone up to 104° F. The pain has moved from around her belly button down to the lower right quadrant of her abdomen. It's very tender about 1/3 of the way between the front of the pelvic crest and the naval (McBurney's) point.

The pain is bringing tears to the patient's eyes.

What do you do, now?

DC:

Hope for the best.

DO or MD:
>
> Operate.
>
> The findings are now classic for appendicitis. The surgery is highly dangerous under the conditions. You could be unnecessarily endangering her life, if your diagnosis is wrong. If, on the other hand, your diagnosis is correct and you do nothing, she will almost certainly die.
>
> It's a tough call. Ultimately, of course, it is the patient's choice.

REAL LIFE:

When I was an in my fourth year of medical school, doing an externship at a hospital, I worked with a resident who looked like a short version of Grizzly Adams. He had long, bushy blond hair and a long blond beard. He was stocky and about 5'5".

As DO's weren't required to do residencies, he had done a one year internship upon finishing medical school and then set out to practice rural medicine in the far off wilderness of Montana. After a few years of practicing in Montana, he came back east, to Iowa, to get some more education and complete a residency in family medicine.

He loved to tell us stories of his medical adventures in the Treasure State. He was the only doctor for a hundred miles and cowboys – yes, real live cowboys - would come to him only when they just couldn't tough-it-out, anymore.

He told of a cowboy who came in with a broken leg. This doctor had only minimal orthopedic training and advised the cowpoke to travel the hundred miles to see an orthopedic surgeon. The result would likely be far better. "Nope," the cowboy answered, "I've gotta get back to work. I don't care how it looks. Just set it so's I can walk on it and that'll be good enough." The doc liked what a tough breed of people these were.

One day, another gentleman came in with what turned out to be a severe appendicitis. There wasn't time to get him to a hospital, even by helicopter. The doctor had to operate immediately. In fact, he was afraid that he was too late or that once he got the patient's belly opened up, the second he touched the appendix, it might burst, releasing bacteria all over the inside of the abdomen thus causing peritonitis.

The doctor had no general anesthesia. All he had was lots of lidocaine (local anesthetic) and some whiskey. He used what he had. He injected lidocaine all over the area of the abdomen where the appendix was likely to be found and gave the cowboy some whiskey to drink – just like in the movies.

As he told it, the operation was a success and the patient survived – much to his complete and utter surprise.

SCENARIO 5

Out on the run, one of your younger group members, a 9 year old boy, gets quite ill. When you first started your journey, the little guy just had a runny nose. It never really got better, but hadn't gotten worse, either. He has a history of allergies, so his mom just figured it was his usual allergic problems acting up. Unfortunately, not long after the group is underway, the boy develops both pains in his face and in his right ear.

You're the doctor. What are your concerns? Is this serious or not? Do you just keep the boy moving with the group or is this something you need to treat? If you choose to treat it, how do you treat it?

Choose your profession:
   a. Chiropractor
   b. Dentist
   c. DO
   d. MD

Your Choice: _____

DC:

As a chiropractor, can you diagnose the child's problem? Probably.

What are you trained to do to treat the boy?

As always, it depends on what school you went to and what experiences you've picked up along the way. Generally speaking, you want the boy to heal up naturally. If you have vitamins and minerals such as zinc, or even some plants which boost immune function to fight off any infection, you can employ those.

Manipulation of the spine and head might actually prove somewhat helpful, as well.

MD:

You can certainly diagnose the problem. You conclude that the boy has most likely developed a bacterial sinusitis due to his poor sinus drainage caused by his chronic allergies. Your concerns are that in children, this can rapidly develop into something very serious. You are aware that kids have little health reserve, so an infection can incapacitate them quickly. A simple ear infection or sinusitis can quickly develop into something far more ominous such as osteomyelitis (infection of the bones, in this case of the jaw or face) or mastoiditis (infection of spaces within the bone behind the ear) if not properly and quickly treated. Sinus infections can also develop into sepsis (body-

wide infection spread within the bloodstream) or even
meningitis (infection of the coverings around the brain
and spinal cord). Most of these more serious
complications can be lethal and should be avoided at
all costs.

As an MD, you select the antibiotic Augmentin™ (if
the child is not allergic to it) and hydration. Keeping
the child's fluid levels up is crucial to recovery.

The child will most likely get better, but what can you
do for his pain? You may not want to give him too
much ibuprofen as it can be very hard on his stomach.
Narcotics are something to try to avoid in younger
kids, if at all possible.

DO

The DO agrees with all the considerations which
would concern an MD. As a DO, you would also
likely choose Augmentin and hydration as a start to
therapy. In addition, however, you may perform OMT
to the child to mobilize their immune system more
effectively. You also have one other tool: cranial
OMT.

Cranial OMT is effective in all age groups, but can be
extremely effective in children whose cranial bones
may not be as fully formed as an adult's. Manipulation
of the cranial bones can open up the sinus drainage
ports, allowing mucus to drain more freely. Continued
hydration can thin the mucus and help it drain more
quickly, as well. Now, that you've given the mucus a
way out, the pressure in the sinuses may get relieved
much more quickly and the infected material will more
likely be quickly eliminated, decreasing both pain and
recovery time with less need for pain relievers.

REAL LIFE:

I've used these techniques for sinus drainage dozens of times on adults and children, alike, with excellent results and, very frequently, with immediate relief of pain.

SCENARIO 6

FINALLY, after weeks of walking, you're lucky enough to find some transportation. Everything is rolling right along (not that you actually know where you're heading, but in the movies, you're always heading somewhere to escape the Zombies.)

Your mechanic, a 50 year-old male who keeps your vehicles running and your guns and other portable equipment operating has, from working so hard on the vehicles and equipment, developed what he believes is severe arthritis in his shoulder. He's always had a little pain, ever since an injury to his shoulder while playing football with his sons several years ago. If he can't use his shoulder, he can't use a wrench and you're all back to walking and living in primitive conditions and in fear.

Over time, the mechanic begins feeling poorly in general, gets flushed in the face, and is getting headaches, regularly. He's been taking ibuprofen to relieve his arthritis pain, but now he's feeling worse.

Choose your profession:
   a. Chiropractor
   b. Dentist
   c. DO
   d. MD

   Your Choice: _____

What are you thinking? What can you do for him?

MD:

As an MD you have been giving your mechanic
Vicodin (narcotic) and ibuprofen (NSAID), because
you have a large supply and need him to keep working.
When his headaches start, you notice that he's
requiring more and more pain relievers to quell his
headaches. You don't want him taking too many
narcotics, so you increase his dosage of ibuprofen.

As far as the shoulder goes, you do some testing and
determine that the rotator cuff (shoulder tendon
complex) is likely injured. You're not detecting any
crepitus (crunchiness) in the shoulder when he moves
it, so you're not really sure it's arthritis. You think he
might also have an injury to a piece of cartilage in the
shoulder, called the glenoid labrum, to which the
biceps muscle attaches. It might be what's called a
SLAP tear.

If it is a SLAP tear and/or a rotator cuff tear, you know
that only surgery can repair it. You are, however,
acutely aware that your diagnosis could be wrong and
it might be arthritic in nature (meaning the bones of the
shoulder would be damaged and not really something
you could surgically repair, under the current primitive
conditions). If you cut his shoulder open and don't
find a tear to repair, you will have exposed him to
injury and infection (which could, of course prove
lethal) for no reason. It's a crying shame you have no
x-ray machines or MRI's with which to take a look at
the shoulder to make the diagnosis before you attempt
the surgery.

You are also aware that it could take months for the
surgery to heal and the mechanic will be unable to use
his arm much during that time, though you are going to
prescribe some intensive therapy. In fact, just because

of the surgery he runs the risk of developing what's known as a "frozen shoulder" which is common after shoulder surgeries. It's an even more painful condition which results from post-surgical scars developing and literally 'freezing' the shoulder, making it impossible to move. A frozen shoulder may prevent him from ever being able to fully use the arm, again.

Can you afford to take that risk?

On the other hand, you are having a major concern that your mechanic might be developing something even worse, such as a brain tumor. That could potentially be causing his headaches, though there are a number of other conditions, most of which are quite serious, which could also be causing his headaches.

As a really good MD you decide to take his blood pressure. It's 190/110 – hypertensive crisis or, as most would say, 'stroke level' (normal blood pressure is <140/90). If you're lucky, you brought a limited supply of medications to control high blood pressure. You give these to your mechanic. It helps his headaches, but you'll soon run out of the medication.

As a good doctor, you suspect the ibuprofen might even be causing the high blood pressure. It's not uncommon for NSAIDs like ibuprofen to affect the kidney which causes a rise in blood pressure.

You take the mechanic off the NSAIDs. Within a day or two, his blood pressure drops way down and his headaches cease. The headaches were caused by the intense high blood pressure.

Unfortunately, his shoulder pain is worse than ever and he's finding it hard to even move his arm.

DC:

As a chiropractor might keep fixing the spine and maybe you even know how to manipulate the shoulder, but if he has a SLAP tear or arthritis, the condition will likely not improve with just manipulation, no matter how good you are.

In addition, how will you know what is causing his headaches? Suppose you even think to take his blood pressure and find out it's stroke level. What does that tell you? How will you treat him? Are you well-versed in the causes of high blood pressure, including that NSAIDs can cause it?

DO:

As a DO you get a complete history and do a complete physical. Your mechanic's temperature is normal. His pulse is slightly fast. Respiratory rate is normal and blood pressure is 190/110. Your physical examination also reveals a likely rotator cuff tear and likely SLAP tear.

What do you do?

As a good DO you immediately take the mechanic off the NSAIDs and administer medication, if you have some, to bring down his high blood pressure in order to prevent a stroke or heart attack.

The blood pressure goes down, the headaches go away and the shoulder pain gets worse than ever.

Are you planning on doing surgery?

NOOOO! Too many risks. You have Prolotherapy* solution and syringes. You opt to inject the shoulder with a mixture of Prolotherapy solution and anesthetic. It will cause the patient's body to react and heal itself in a relatively short time – and you don't run much of a risk of infection and really no risk of a frozen shoulder.

ANALYSIS:
What happened?

All medicines are poisons if either used for the wrong reasons or in too large an amount or too often. Just like chiropractors, all DO's are taught that ALL MEDICINES ARE POISONS. The difference between chiropractic, which consequently decided that virtually no medicines should ever be used, is that in osteopathic medicine we are taught to weigh the benefits vs. the risks when deciding whether or not to use a medication. Ibuprofen is a wonderful drug for many things. It does, however, have some potential downsides: it can cause stomach ulcers and can affect kidneys which can cause high blood pressure, in some people. It should be used in moderation and when appropriate, not used like candy.

The mechanic almost had a stroke due to the high BP which was due to the effect of the NSAIDs on his kidneys. Pain could be better and more safely controlled by Morphine, but most doctors have been taught to be afraid of it because of its addictive potential. This is wrong, but that's a story for another book.

Osteopathy is all about BALANCE. You balance the patient's needs with their desire for treatment. You carefully select appropriate treatments and medications balancing the risks of treating and the benefits of treating versus the risks of not treating. When it comes to selecting medications, you select the one(s) with the greatest potential benefit and the fewest risks, whenever possible. You always try to use the fewest medications or the lowest dosages necessary to achieve your treatment goals in order to minimize risk to the patient.

The idea that "if a little is good, more is better" is NOT a good concept in medicine.

*Prolotherapy is also known by several other names including Sclerotherapy and 'Stimulated Ligament Reconstruction'. Prolotherapy consists of injecting an 'irritant solution', usually of something that is not even a medication, but can be as simple as dextrose (a sugar) and water into a ligament or tendon. The body recognizes this irritation and is fooled into believing there is a new injury. The body responds with inflammation.

Inflammation, contrary to popular belief, is actually very, very useful. Inflammation is the mechanism by which the body heals from infection and wounds. CHRONIC inflammation is not useful. In fact, prolonged inflammation is damaging to tissues and can lead to weakening of ligaments and tendons. Acute (short-term) inflammation, however, as in response to a new injury - is healing.

Acute inflammation results in the opening of blood vessels around the injured area, resulting in increased blood flow – bringing more oxygen, nutrients, and healing white blood cells to the area. Some of the white cells fight infection. Others, called fibroblasts, lay down new fibrous connective tissue. These new layers strengthen and heal damaged ligaments and tendons and can even help regenerate damaged cartilage, thus reducing arthritis. Pain is ultimately reduced and often completely eliminated when Prolotherapy is properly utilized.

Both MD's and DO's use Prolotherapy. It was, in fact, first discovered by an MD. In the US, today, however, in my experience, a significantly higher percentage of DO's use or recommend Prolotherapy than do MD's.

I have used Prolotherapy on and off for many years. I always recommend it when I deem it appropriate. I have even undergone Prolotherapy treatment, myself, for chronic back pain, with excellent results.

REAL LIFE:

The case, above, is based on a real-life case of someone very close to me. As a young woman, approximately 6 years before we met, my friend had fallen on some ice. Her feet went out from under her and she fell backwards, her arms outstretched behind her to break her fall.

For months afterwards, she had terrible whole upper-body pain. No one found anything wrong with her.

The upper-body pain eventually subsided. During the next two years, however, she began developing severe spasms in her arms, back, and shoulders. The muscles would develop into multiple distinct knots, easily palpated. No cause was ever found.

Because her doctors could not figure out the cause, she was eventually sent to a chiropractor. The chiropractor cracked her back, trying to help. As a result of the treatment, however, the pain was so horribly intensified the she was sent to the ER, the next day, where they tested her for a heart attack. The results were negative, meaning her heart was fine. The pain became so intense, though, that narcotic pain relievers couldn't even begin to alleviate it.

She was eventually sent for other tests. She received x-rays and an MRI of her upper body, including her shoulders. The radiologists told her she had a bone spur in her shoulder which might be causing the pain.

She had an EMG (electrically active needles inserted into muscles and nerves in the arm, back and neck to measure muscle and nerve activity). The neurologist told her that her carpal tunnel syndrome (which usually causes pain and numbness only in the hand) was the cause of her arm pain.

It was ALL WRONG. These doctors had no clue what the problem was.

When we finally met, my friend was experiencing fairly constant bilateral shoulder pain and knotty spasms in her arms. Her right arm was far worse than her left. I started performing manipulation and western acupuncture on her and things began to slowly change. We peeled off layers of pain. Eventually, much of her pain was reduced, but my physical diagnosis showed that she likely had SLAP tears in each shoulder. She didn't want corrective surgery, though.

I also noted that her breast bone (which is actually made up of three parts, not one) was injured so that the top bone was overlapping the one beneath it. I admit it was a difficult diagnosis – and fairly rare, which is why no one was looking for it. Still, this appeared to be a major contributor to her pain. Whenever I could get the bones properly aligned, the knots in her arms and most of her pain would disappear. Unfortunately, the bones didn't stay aligned for more than three days at a time, and sometimes for as little as a few hours.

Eventually, she also developed a completely different type of left shoulder pain, so severe that she almost couldn't move her arm. I diagnosed a rotator cuff tear – torn tendons of the muscles which move the shoulder.

It should be noted that none of this required any x-rays or MRI's. With good osteopathic and physical diagnostic skills and good history-taking skills, I was able to deduce her injuries without the assistance of technology. Of course, once we sent her to her regular doctor, he ordered an MRI of her left shoulder, again. Guess what was found: a SLAP tear of the glenoid labrum and an 80% tear of her rotator cuff. She was immediately offered surgery.

Fortunately for my friend, she had recently had thyroid surgery. That surgery, however, was complicated by pneumonia which put her back in the hospital for a longer stay than she'd had for the original surgery. I say 'fortunately' because having had a recent surgery and then a serious complication, she refused any further surgeries.

Instead, I convinced her to try Prolotherapy for her shoulder injuries. Only a week after her very first prolo treatment, she reported that her pain level was reduced 35-40% and the shoulder was much more mobile.

IVAN
An Osteopath is a doctor for people. Turn around.

(Isaac [stooped crookedly] does as he's told. Ivan gets him in a full-Nelson.)

IVAN
Breathe in . . . out . . . in . . . out.

Ivan lifts Isaac off the ground adjusting every vertebra in his back. There is a ripple of cracks. Isaac stands up straight, much straighter than before. He holds his head high. A mild hush goes through the crowd.

ISAAC
Thank you!

IVAN
Don't mention it. Anyone else has a problem, come to me. In fact, you can just think of me as "The Great Healer."

SCENARIO 7

After a week of driving unpaved roads and around highway wrecks (it's awfully hard to move down highways clogged by abandoned vehicles and dead people while trying to avoid the main arteries where the Zombies congregate) your gas reserves are almost depleted. It's time to stop riding and start walking, again. Unfortunately, however, while getting out of the cool, souped-up, low-to-the ground little sportster he was driving, the leader of your small band of refugees – who's been under just a bit of stress since this whole thing started – suddenly gets severe, debilitating low back pain, nearly in the buttock, so sharp that he can neither get into nor out of the vehicle and is stuck half-way in.

Choose your profession:
     a. Chiropractor
     b. Dentist
     c. DO
     d. MD

Your Choice: _____

What's wrong with him? What can you do for him?

MD:

My experience is that MD's generally have no idea what to do with this type of injury. They give the patient pain relievers and muscle relaxants and hope the pain may more or less resolve within 10 days or so. They love to get x-rays and MRI's of such injuries, though. They seem to always think the patient will be relieved to know that 'nothing was found.'

I don't know about you, but when my body tells me something is severely wrong and you tell me 'nothing was found,' I tend to lose confidence in you and your ability to help me with this problem and with future medical problems. Something is obviously wrong. YOU, Mr. MD, may not have found it, but it's there.

Perhaps the MD could even inject some lidocaine, but even if it works a little, when the anesthetic wears off, the pain will return full force and your leader will become incapacitated, again.

Your choices will be to use the gurney to push him on (which will still be mightily painful for him, I promise), stay where you are for a week or more and hope he's able to walk by then, or leave him for Zombie-bait.

DC:

A chiropractor would almost certainly recognize what happened, almost immediately. This is a classic example of how the sacroiliac joint gets stuck.

The sacrum is an upside-down triangle of bone which sits in your very low back nestled between the two parts of the pelvis, just above your natal or intergluteal cleft (okay, fine: butt-crack). The spine sits on top of the sacrum's base.

Trust me, this pain is among the most severe a person can ever experience. Its intensity can be paralyzing.

When the pain is this severe, however, although the chiropractor may know how to treat it, the 'cracking' techniques generally won't work. The patient's pain is simply so severe, the area is so "hot," that it can't be handled with anything more than the gentlest touch. No 'cracking' techniques can be used.

A chiropractor well-versed in a variety of softer techniques can likely perform some manipulations which could easily relieve the pain almost immediately. If they are not well-versed in such techniques, sometimes manipulating the spine above the area of pain can be enough to start the healing process so that the pain will resolve in a matter of days.

DO:

Knowing the history, a good DO should suspect the mechanism of injury, just like the chiropractor. Unlike the chiropractor, however, as a DO you can give your fearless leader pain medication and muscle relaxants, if you feel they will help. You can also inject lidocaine into the joint but, unlike the MD, your purpose is not just to temporarily relieve the pain. The reason for giving the anesthetic is to reduce the pain so that you can more effectively perform OMM directly to the sacrum and pelvis. If you do this, the patient will likely be able to walk reasonably well within a day or so (maybe immediately). More importantly, the severe pain should not return and any residual pain should be easily controlled by the oral pain medications you have available and should completely resolve within a couple of days.

No bait left for the Zombies, today.

REAL LIFE:

I've diagnosed and treated this particular injury many, many times in my career. I've been called into the office at 10 pm at night to fix a patient and I've even taught osteopathic undergraduate classes how to recognize the injury by history and diagnosis and how to treat it.

When I was an intern working in the emergency room, I handled things quite a bit differently than my MD colleagues. I could even treat things that my attendings (overseeing physician teachers) couldn't do – but only because they had never been trained.

In a single month in the ER in a little hospital in the little town of Coldwater, Michigan we had not one, not even two, but three cases like this come in to the ER. Each time, I asked to take the case. These patients came in on wheelchairs and on gurneys. Usually, they were moaning in pain with tears running down their faces. When I went to examine them, sometimes they screamed, just from being touched.

I didn't need x-rays to tell me what was wrong. I listened to how they got injured. I did a good physical examination including an osteopathic hands-on examination and easily diagnosed the problem. In every case, I performed manipulation and these patients who had been wheeled in to the emergency department walked out under their own power.

My attendings always expressed amazement. They'd NEVER SEEN ANYBODY WALK OUT of the ER after such an injury. "How did you do it?" They'd ask.

Perhaps my proudest moment as an intern was when one of my attending physicians, an MD and a veteran of more than 20 years in emergency care, came to me after such a case (he'd personally seen me handle two of the cases) and said, "If we can ever find the time, you have got to teach me how you do that!"

Somehow, I didn't think I would be able to teach him in 5 minutes what it had taken me 4 years to learn.

BIZZY (Human born into the world of the Alien Apocalypse) speaking with IVAN:
(confused)
"Are you an alien? You don't look like one."

IVAN
(shakes his head)
No. I'm from Earth. I'm a doctor.

BIZZY
(nods again)
Oh. What's a doctor?

IVAN
You don't know what a doctor is?

BIZZY
(shakes her head)
Uh-uh.

IVAN
I help people.

BIZZY
(nods)
How sweet.

SCENARIO 8

Okay, you've been primed. Let's see if you've learned anything:

One of the women tends the few small children in your group. This is a vital job for several reasons, but perhaps most importantly – these young ones may be the last hope of mankind. They must be looked after, fed, cleansed, taught, and kept safe. If this woman can't do her job, someone else who has another important job may have to do it. You're a small, mobile community and everyone contributes to the best of their ability.

This evening, after a particularly stressful day with the kids (little Sally had gone off into the woods to relieve herself and disappeared for 2 hours) this bedraggled, hard-working woman was out looking for firewood for the dinner fire. She was bent low several minutes, picking up kindling and small logs. Suddenly, she went to stand up when, "AHHH!" she couldn't straighten up. She had terrible back pain on the right. It ran from her low (lumbar) spine out toward her hip.

Choose your profession:
- a. Chiropractor
- b. PT (Physical Therapist)
- c. DO
- d. MD

Your Choice: _____

Do you think it could be her sacroiliac joint causing her pain?

[NEXT PAGE]

NOOOO! It's not her sacroiliac joint!

Well, at least you were paying SOME attention.

Bending over and straightening up can cause sacroiliac problems. If you paid careful attention to the history, however, you would have noticed that the pain was not way down in her back just above her buttocks. The pain is higher than that and more to the right side than toward the center.

What can you do for her?

DC:

> As a chiropractor, you believe the woman may have either a lumbar vertebral subluxation (chiropractic speak for a malfunctioning vertebra) or a herniated lumbar disc. Since the woman really doesn't have neurologic signs (no numbness, no muscle weakness, normal reflexes) you feel that a disc herniation is less likely. You manipulate her back.

> Unfortunately, there is only very minor improvement. She still can't stand up straight and leans to the right.

MD:

> As an MD, you come to the same conclusion as the chiropractor. Since you don't know (and may not even 'believe' in manipulation), however, you simply offer her some pain medications and muscle relaxants, tell her to rest and hope the pain improves by tomorrow.

> She says, "Fine. And if it doesn't improve by tomorrow, YOU take care of the kids and gather the firewood."

PT:

As a physical therapist, you don't actually try to make a diagnosis. You just know that if you have manipulative skills, you use them. If that doesn't work, you work at exercising the patient. Of course, you have no exercise equipment with you, so you have to improvise. Unfortunately, all the exercise in the world won't have this lady back on her feet by tomorrow. In fact, although it may eventually help her, it never gets her completely better and the pain keeps coming back. She's never quite the same.

DO:

As a DO, you think about the history she relates to you. Then you do a **good physical exam**. You agree it's not likely to be a disc. It may, in fact, be a vertebral malfunction. You do some manipulation, but not just to the lumbar spine. You also manipulate the sacrum, to take pressure off the lumbar spine and manipulate the thoracic (chest) spine for the same reason. If you're really good, you manipulate the pelvis and cervical (neck) spine, as well, as these have connections that can cause lumbar pain.

Unfortunately, the woman's pain is not much improved and you're dreading having to chase after those kids, tomorrow. Desperate, you rethink how she was injured, the fact that she's bent to the right, and the fact that your spinal manipulation failed to help her much. That's when the lightbulb goes off.

You gingerly grab hold of the right side of her back about 3 inches from the spine and she yelps. You've just found out that she has a quadratus lumborum muscle spasm. (The quadratus lumborum (QL) is a fairly large muscle on either side of the spine which attaches to the pelvis, the upper four lumbar vertebrae and to the 12th (lower-most) rib.)

You've already treated the lumbar and thoracic spine and the pelvis. Now, you know to additionally treat the ribs, especially the 12th rib. You finish up by doing a stretch very specific to the quadratus lumborum muscle.

The patient has instant relief. You will not be chasing children, tomorrow, unless you want to.

REAL LIFE:

Story 1:

In my many years of practice, I have found QL spasms are one of the most commonly missed causes of acute and chronic pain. Actually, when the spasm lasts for years (yes, YEARS), it becomes quite permanent and is no longer called a spasm. At that point, the permanent spasm has caused fibrous adhesions to develop within the muscle that help hold the muscle in the shortened (contracted) state. It is then called a 'contracture'.

I have come across many cases of fairly acute QL spasms that were missed by both Chiropractors and other doctors. When fresh, they're relatively easy to treat. When older and developed into contractures, they're somewhat more difficult, but not impossible to treat. It just takes a little longer.

I have had not one, but two very interesting cases in my career of people who have had QL contractures. One of them was in her mid-twenties when we met. She gave me the history that when she was 15, she'd been working in a cramped attic space and had been bent over for hours. When she came out, she was unable to completely straighten up.

She had been to numerous doctors and even chiropractors over the years. No one had ever been able to diagnose her pain nor help it. Until recently, she hadn't even been able to sleep comfortable or very long, at night. Only a few months before we met, though, she had bought an electronic hospital-style bed which she could fold up – lifting her legs and upper body so she was folded into a 'V' shape; it was the most comfortable way for her to sleep. She had finally taken to using marijuana, medicinally, to help with the pain and to help her sleep at night.

The history, alone, including the mechanism of injury and the way she folded herself up at night made me suspicious of a QL contracture. Still, I did a <u>full neurological and musculoskeletal examination to make certain I wasn't missing anything</u>. I ended up treating her, including doing specific treatments for the spine, pelvis, ribs, and QL, as outlined above. Her pain was reduced by 60% or more after a single treatment.

Story 2:

There was a second patient who had been in pain for 16 full years. He couldn't tell me exactly how he injured himself, so my antennae weren't up, enough. He told me that he'd been to the chiropractor every week or two for YEARS. The chiropractic treatments helped, sometimes for a few hours. Sometimes they helped for a few days, but the pain always returned. No matter what I did, though, I just couldn't seem to reproduce his pain which would have helped me pinpoint the cause.

I was puzzled (I must have been tired, that day) and couldn't figure out why he was having what he described as lumbar (low back) pain. Finally, without fixing him, I let him leave the examining room.

I sat at my desk, writing up the results of our session, brows furrowed, with something niggling at the back of my mind. I'd seen this, before, but I couldn't put my finger on it.

BAM!! It hit me.

I literally rushed out of my office, grabbed the patient from the receptionist and made him return to the examining room. I grabbed hold of his quadratus lumborum muscle and he said, "That's it! That's my pain."

It helps to know what you're looking for.

SCENARIO 9

"I can't do it. I can't walk, anymore. My leg just hurts too damn much." He sits down on a log and raises his left leg onto the log.

One of your company, a 68 year old retired lawyer has been complaining for the last 2 days. He just told a couple of people that his leg 'hurt', but he kept going. This is the first you've heard about it.

"Let me see your leg," you say.

He tries to pull his pant leg up, but he can't. There really isn't any modesty when you're running for your life; he stands up, unbuckles his belt and drops his trousers to the ground.

His left lower leg is at least three times as big as his right.

"Whoa!" says a smart-aleck 14 year old (your lone teenager in the group). "What is THAT?"

You examine the leg and get the man's history. He has no history of swelling (edema) of his legs, in the past. He has no heart conditions or respiratory problems. He has no high blood pressure. No kidney problems. In fact, he's been remarkably healthy and took no medicines before the Zombie Apocalypse other than some vitamins and a daily baby aspirin. He's always been extremely active, physically. He did travel to Asia about three years ago, with his wife, before she passed away. He remembers catching his foot in a hole in the dark a couple of nights ago, when he went to relieve himself. It hurt his knee, but only for a minute or so. He has no fever and does not recall any recent infections. He's never had tuberculosis and was married to the same woman for 43 years – until the Zombies got her.

Your general physical exam is unremarkable except for the enlarged leg which is obviously full of fluid. The leg is not hot and shows no sign of redness or infection.

Choose your profession:
    a.   Chiropractor
    b.   Dentist
    c.   DO
    d.   MD

        Your Choice: _____

What are the potential diagnoses? I'll give you some:
    1.   Elephantiasis – a disease common in Africa and Asia. It is caused by a filarial worm (lymphatic filariasis) which ends up blocking the lymphatic system. As a result, fluids back up into places like the limbs or scrotum. The affected areas can become many times their normal size.
    2.   Congestive heart failure – the heart gets over-stressed and can stop pumping with enough pressure to force the fluids from the feet back up the veins to the heart. The fluid ends up seeping out of the veins and into the surrounding tissues, causing edema (swelling).

3. A number of other infectious diseases such as lymphogranuloma venereum (a sexually transmitted bacterial infection) or tuberculosis could cause a similar presentation.
4. Injury.

DC:

As a chiropractor, you may be partially correct in doing spinal manipulation to improve neurologic function of the leg. There may be other benefits such as improved immune function and improved blood flow. Depending upon your training, you may direct some specific treatment toward the leg, itself. These general benefits could prove quite helpful, especially in the event that the process is an infectious or circulatory problem (related to blood flow).

MD:

As an MD, you will likely be looking for causes such as heart disease, elephantiasis, or other bacterial infections although I'm hard-pressed to see how you'll do it without technology. You have no methods for improving blood flow or immunity. You don't even have a microscope to take a blood or tissue sample to see if you can see bacteria or filarial worms. There's not much you can do other than a trial of antibiotics. The Bactrim might work against lymphogranuloma venereum, but you have nothing which could treat filariasis or TB. Maybe you would even consider some kind of surgery as a last resort?

SMART ALECK TEENAGER:

You would like to throw the lawyer out as Zombie bait and keep moving.

LAWYER:

You would like to throw the teenager out as Zombie bait and get some peace and quiet.

DO:
Although it does cross your mind that an attorney
might make excellent Zombie bait, you also realize that
we will need lawyers and judges to re-establish the rule
of law, should the Zombies ever die off, allowing
civilization to once again assert itself.

As a result, you actually desire to keep the attorney
alive and safe from the clutches of Zombie-kind. The
teenager, on the other hand …

You hope he will learn and mature before you all
decide that Zombies would find him tender and
delicious.

As an osteopathic physician, you consider the
possibilities. You and an MD would both realize that
lymphogranuloma venereum is unlikely because of the
patient's long-standing monogamous relationship.
Both TB and Elephantiasis are possibilities, but even if
he has one of them, you have no effective medications
for treating either disease. If he has either, he's in
trouble.

You consider the possibility of congestive heart failure,
but you don't think it's very likely. Normally, though
not always, congestive heart failure causes BOTH legs
to swell. It would be fairly rare see it cause only one
leg to swell, especially to twice normal size, without
the other leg being affected, at all.

Maybe his stepping in a hole has something to do with
it. You decide to do a trial of conservative therapy, i.e.
OMT – to the thoracic inlet/outlet (upper part of the
chest, including the clavicles), cisterna chyle (a major
part of the lymphatic system), some stretching of
tissues of the low back, pelvis, and lower extremity
(especially around the knee) to open both venous and

lymphatic flow. You make sure the ankle and fibular head are back where they belong.

You know that the venous and lymphatic systems are low pressure systems which don't work well if they are kinked or are getting squeezed between sheets of tightened tissues or muscles. You do some OMT called lymphatic pumps. All of this is directed to opening up the pathways of lymphatic flow and encouraging fluids to return from the tissues where they don't belong back into the bloodstream.

You figure that if you can make it easier for the lymph to return to the blood circulation, the swelling should go down. If it doesn't work, you've lost nothing. You still have the less conservative options open to you such as a trial of antibiotics or even surgery, if the leg starts to show signs of deterioration such as gangrene.

If it does work, you save your meager store of antibiotics for the future, prevent unnecessary surgery, save the patient's leg and maybe his life.

The teenager is disappointed.

REAL LIFE:

When I was in my residency, I had a case just like this. An older woman who was already a patient of mine, who was otherwise fairly healthy with no history of heart disease, travel, or infection presented to my office with only her left leg swollen.

My physical exam revealed no specific cause, so I did a trial of OMT as described, above. The swelling in her leg was gone within minutes.

Dr. IVAN HOOD, osteopathic physician, just returned from 40 years in space to a desolate-looking world but before he learns that it is overrun by giant termite-like aliens:

"...the way I've got it worked out is that my services are going to be at a high premium. In fact, Osteopaths will be in greater demand than M.D.s. My newest theory is that the future is utopia for everyone, excluding M.D.s, of course, and I will be known as "The Great Healer."

Aida [his companion]:
(snorts) "Ha!"

IVAN:
What's the matter, you don't think I have the potential?

AIDA
"I don't think it matters what you think! Nothing ever works out the way it's supposed to ... I think we're all breathing high levels of radiation and we'll all be dead by nightfall."

SCENARIO 10

Now, you've done it. You've run smack into a nest of hungry Zombies. Your group heads for the shallow river you crossed a little ways back. Everyone knows Zombies won't cross the water!

Just as you reach the river, the Zombies catch up. Your huntress and a fellow with a shotgun have stayed slightly behind to fight off the Zombie horde so that the children and elderly can get in the water, first. Your two heroes are unable to kill all the Zombies, but stop most of them.

Just as the two are about to jump into the water, themselves, an injured Zombie crawls up and bites the shotgun wielder on the leg. Your hero bats at the Zombie's head with the back of his now empty shot gun and sends the creature flying.

The Huntress, catching the action out of the corner of her eye, turns and sends a crossbow bolt straight through Mr. Zombie's eye socket ... then she screams in pain.

A Zombie has snuck up behind her and bitten her on the muscle between her neck and shoulder. Before he can take a second bite, she reels around, catching him under the jaw with her Bowie knife ... which just makes the attacker pause for a second and step back. That's enough space for her fellow survivor, who has quickly reloaded his shotgun, to explode the Zombie's head with buckshot.

The two heroes jump into the water, hurriedly wade across, and scramble up the other bank.

The Zombies moan in frustration, but you are all safe for the moment.

Sort of.

You now have two injured compatriots, one bitten on the leg, the other bitten on the shoulder.

Choose your profession:
        a.   Chiropractor
        b.   Dentist
        c.   DO
        d.   MD

        Your Choice: _____

What's your next step?

It doesn't matter what kind of doctor you are, you can apply good first-aid principles. Cleanse the wounds with a hefty dose of soap and water, especially water ... lots and lots of sterile water. Try to wash out as much of the infecting bacteria as possible.

In the case of your shotgun wielder, you might want to consider a tourniquet of the leg until you can decide what to do. This might stop bacteria from traveling up the blood stream and infecting the rest of his body.

Obviously, no such measures can be taken for your huntress. You bandage her neck wound. When both people are stabilized, you need to consider ...

What's your next step?

[NEXT PAGE]

DC:

You can offer them both hydration (not IV) and chiropractic manipulation. Improving the body's ability to heal itself by improving neural flow from the spine definitely couldn't hurt and may have substantial benefit.

Other than that, it's watch and wait. Keep them comfortable. Give them oxygen when they start to have severe respiratory symptoms. If they survive the respiratory failure stage, they may completely recover. If either dies of the respiratory illness, your group will need to burn the body immediately as the victim will resurrect within six hours with a ravenous appetite for human flesh.

MD:

In addition to the conservative measures, above, you have some additional options. You can hydrate the victims with IV fluids, if they become unable to drink. You know that antibiotics won't stop the Zombism bacteria, but you might decide to administer some antibiotics, anyway, to prevent infection from other, less exotic bacteria, that the Zombie bites may carry. It would be a shame to have the victims survive the Zombie illness only to succumb to an infection from a bacteria that could have been treated with the medicines you have on hand. A still more conservative approach would be to wait and observe, treating with antibiotics only at the first sign of wound infection. Both approaches make sense, really.

For the man with the bite on his leg, you might further consider immediate amputation to attempt to prevent spread of the Zombism bacteria to the rest of the body. If you've tourniqueted the leg, that might be a reasonable option. Discuss it with your patient.

DO:

        Same options as above. In addition, you would likely
want to treat the body with OMT to enhance blood
flow and lymphatic function. The more capable the
body is of mounting a strong immune response, the
more likely it is that the victim will be able to eradicate
the bacteria before he or she succumbs to the disease.

***

The leg-bite victim opts not to have the amputation. He's
philosophical about it. "If it's my time, it's my time," he says.
"I might even die from surgical complications and the woods
are kind of a dirty place to perform a surgery. Just do
everything you can to stop the infection and keep me
comfortable, Doc. Without my leg, I'd just become a burden to
everyone, anyway. I don't think I'd want to live that way."

You comply with the patient's wishes. Now, it's watch and
wait for both of the patients. You make camp and prepare for
what's coming.

***

Sure enough, within two days, both bite victims start to show
signs of lung problems. They don't cough, but find it harder
and harder to take in a deep breath. Their muscles are
beginning to cramp and neither is able to be up and around.
Within a short time, neither has the strength to talk, eat, or
drink. They are lying listless upon their makeshift beds. Each
has a fever of more than 102°F and is complaining of a
headache.

What do you do next?

[NEXT PAGE]

DC:

> Keep them comfortable. Manipulate their spines. Perhaps you know some other techniques to help with respiration. You apply those. Unfortunately, the man is very much against alternative type medicines. As philosophical as he is, he will not let you do manipulation on him.

MD:

> You start IV hydration. If you have some dextrose (sugar) IV solution, you provide it to give some energy to fight the disease process.
>
> Perhaps you provide some acetaminophen or ibuprofen to reduce the patients' fevers and keep them more comfortable. If the pain gets severe enough, you give them Vicodin™ (a combination of hydrocodone [a narcotic pain reliever] and acetaminophen) or morphine to ease their pain.
>
> You have no conflict with the male bite-victim. You don't know how to do any manipulation, anyway.

DO:

> Start IV hydration and dextrose, if available. Do manipulation – not just of the spine, but everywhere you deem appropriate to improve immune function and blood flow, for the huntress. You respect the man's right to refuse your manipulative treatment. You have no choice while he's conscious and able to make sound decisions.
>
> You do not, however, offer acetaminophen, ibuprofen, or Vicodin™ to reduce the fever or relieve the headaches. No, you're not being sadistic.
>
> The headaches might be due to the fever. Reducing the fever could conceivably easily get rid of the headaches. As an osteopathic physician, however, you are aware

that fever is one of the body's methods of fighting infection. Although it may be uncomfortable, a higher body temperature can slow the growth and multiplication of bacteria. You will only treat the fever if it gets so high that it begins to endanger the patient's own proteins (approximately 105-106°F).

Instead of the other choices, you give the patients straight morphine to help control their pain. Morphine does not interfere with the body's immunologic response the way the other medicines do.

***

As the disease progresses, both the huntress' and her companion victim's symptoms are worsening, though the man seems to be getting more severe symptoms more quickly. Eventually, you put both of them on oxygen. Finally, the man becomes unconscious and unarousable.

What do you do next?

[NEXT PAGE]

DC:

You're a terrible human being: you disregard the man's wishes and begin your particular form of manipulation. At least the community supports your decision. If there were law, that would be another matter. Still, you must follow your conscience.

The huntress, without IV hydration, has also become unconscious, despite your best efforts.

In three more days, both are dead.

Prepare the pyres.

MD:

You continue to watch and wait. Both victims are soon unconscious and respirations are becoming shallower and less effective with each passing minute. You know the end is near.

Prepare the pyres.

DO:

You're still a terrible human being and begin manipulation on the man. It seems too little, too late, however. His breathing becomes shallower and less effective. You know his end is near. Prepare the pyre.

Your huntress, on the other hand, is holding steady. With IV hydration and dextrose for energy and regular manipulation, especially lymphatic pumps and rib-raises (to help the patient take deeper breaths), the patient appears to be fighting the disease.

5 days after the Zombie attack, the man is dead and his carcass is ashes.

The huntress, however, appears to be very slightly improving. After another 5 days, she is able to breathe without oxygen or assistance. (That's GREAT, because your oxygen supply is exhausted.) It takes another 2 weeks, but finally she is back on her feet, hunting and protecting your community.

REAL LIFE:

In the Spanish Flu epidemic of 1918-19, between 21 and 30 million people perished, mostly of respiratory complications. It is currently believed that the majority of deaths may not have been due directly to the viral infection, but rather due to secondary bacterial infections (pneumonia) which resulted from compromised bronchial and lung function.

Historical records of medical, osteopathic, and chiropractic treatment provided to patients afflicted with the Spanish Flu show a vast improvement of survival for those treated with either chiropractic care or osteopathic care compared to those treated with only allopathic care. There are a number of methodological problems with the retrospective studies which were performed after the epidemic passed. Many authors have readily pointed them out. Despite this, I have seen no claims from any reliable source that the main point of the studies is inaccurate: **manipulation is very helpful and was likely crucial to patient survival**.

The studies generally showed that approximately 30-40% of people infected with the Spanish Flu ultimately died under allopathic (MD) medical care. On the other hand far fewer (on the order of 0.25% - 1%) of those treated with osteopathic or chiropractic techniques died over the same time period.[11]

In the scenario above, the major reason that osteopathic medicine was superior to chiropractic is the consideration that the patient quickly became dehydrated (which we said was part of the Zombism disease process) and used up her energy reserves so that she was unable to continue her struggling respiratory efforts. Without the use of IV fluids, I speculate that she is less likely to survive as the mucus plugs which develop (see 'Rules Governing Zombism', section III.3.c for details) are more likely to be thinned out by the additional of fluid, making them easier to cough out. This would likely prevent suffocation as well as the creation of airless pockets where secondary bacteria (which thrive in such airless environments) can thrive, which would cause additional complications such as pneumonia.

I'm sure there are those who will disagree, but I believe it is a reasonable conclusion: Do you choose to provide the patient the fullest opportunity to survive or do you adhere to dogma which prevents the use of all good and available methods to assist the patient?

A wounded man spots Ivan and his companions, Bizzy and Alex:

WOUNDED MAN
(groaning)
[Believing Ivan and his companions to be hostile, he says:] Just make it quick, will ya?

(Ivan turns him over and inspects the wound. The guy has a bullet in his side. [He knows he has to remove the bullet or the wounded man could die.] Ivan turns to Bizzy.)

IVAN
Have you got a knife?

(Bizzy reaches into her pack and pulls out a large Bowie Knife. She hands it to Ivan. The wounded guy shuts his eyes tightly expecting death any moment. Ivan looks at Alex and Bizzy.)

IVAN

I don't suppose we have anything antiseptic with us, do we?

(They both shrug. They don't know what he means.)

IVAN
Alcohol?

(Bizzy nods, reaches into her pack and removes a small clay jug. She offers it to Ivan.)

BIZZY
Potato liquor.

IVAN
That'll do.
(he takes a slug and winces [because it tastes *terrible*!])
Smooth.
(he holds it out to the patient)
Here. Drink this.

The wounded guy opens one eye.

WOUNDED MAN
Huh?

IVAN
Drink it. It'll kill the pain.

WOUNDED MAN
Why do you want me to drink that if you're gonna stick me with a knife?

IVAN
I'm a sadist. ...

SCENARIO 11

You've been on the run for weeks, now. You've decided that it's best to stay away from population centers as that would be the most likely place to encounter a large Zombie population. Long ago, your group decided it would be in your best interests to head for unpopulated land – a rural area where the likelihood of encountering hordes of Zombies would be extremely low.

Ideally, you've been searching for an intact, but abandoned farm. You hope to be able to build defenses to protect yourselves, but more importantly, you need a place to start growing your own food. You've been heading south toward warmer climes, so that you will hopefully have a longer growing season. Unfortunately, none of you really knows much about farming beyond growing a backyard garden full of tomatoes and cucumbers which you always had to give away because you didn't even know how to preserve them by canning. Oh, well, you'll figure it all out, right?

Oh ... and you don't exactly have any seeds with you to plant, either.

LUCK!

You city-folk come across the perfect farmhouse in the middle of nowhere, seemingly abandoned – yet with corn and some kind of beans growing all around it. You even hear a soft mooing and "baa" not far off. In addition, there seems to be smaller plots of ... you got it ... tomatoes and cucumbers and even some herbs your city eyes don't recognize, growing closer to the house.

You creep up quietly, wary of potential zombies. Suddenly, an elderly woman appears at the door. This sweetheart of a grandma has a loaded double-barreled shotgun aimed right at your head.

"What d'you want?!" she politely inquires, cocking the first of two hammers.

You stutter as your bowels turn to jelly.

You're hungry. You're thirsty. You're tired. You could really use a shower – and, looking at the gun only 2 feet from your face, your bladder has this sudden urge to empty itself.

The lady whose chest pain you fixed at the beginning of your long journey, your huntress, sees what's happening and quickly intervenes. "We're just looking for a place to stay. We don't mean any harm – at least if you're not a Zombie."

"Actually," the man whose pseudoasthma you cured, interjects (yep, he's still alive without his medications!), "To be honest, we thought this place was abandoned. We were hoping to settle down and maybe set up a community. You know, do some farming and stay alive until this Zombie epidemic passes."

She cocks an eye at the young man (while keeping both barrels pointed at your head, of course). "Abandoned? You city folk think this food grew itself?" Everyone looks around and then at one another, a little embarrassed. Except you, of course. You have both eyes focused inside the gun barrels in front of you. "Food like this doesn't grow itself. It's got to be planted and tended."

The cows moo louder.

"And ya think them cows and sheep been just hidin' in the barn all this time? They got to be cared for. You city folk don't know nothin' about farming, do ya?"

That's when it hits all of you: without somebody who actually knows what they're doing, you have about as much chance of farming successfully as the Pilgrims did their first year at Plymouth.

"You've been running this whole farm by yourself?" the huntress asks, incredulous.

"Heck no. I don't know much about the farming. I do the canning and milking. My husband does the farming."

"Could we talk with him?" the young man asks.

Grandma looks a bit worried, but tries to hide it. "He, uh, ain't feelin' too good, just now."

You can tell it's more than that. Something's seriously wrong. "M-m-maybe I can help," you finally stammer, "I'm a doctor."

She gives you a steely eye, "You ain't a veterinarian, are ya?"

"Not exactly," you squeak out.

***

At long last, the stand-off is over and Grandma takes you to see her husband. Lying in his bed – actually tied down to his bed – is an elderly man, still strong-looking for his years. He doesn't seem to notice that you're even there, though. His eyes wander and he's mumbling to himself. He looks gaunt.

"How long has he been like this," you ask, fearing the worst.

"Only about 2 days," responds the old woman. "Three days ago he was out feedin' the animals and tendin' the farm. Next thing I know, I find him wanderin' 'round like he doesn't know where he is or even who he is. I tied him to the bed just to keep him from wandering off. I thought maybe he had a stroke or maybe he's turnin' into one of those Zombie-things."

You study this poor man, but your thoughts are not only on him. You and your companions realize your best chance for successfully learning to farm and becoming self-sustaining regarding your food supply rests with this elderly gentleman and his wife. You've got to keep him alive and get him back to his former self or you haven't a chance.

CHOICES:

Choose your profession:
  a. Chiropractor
  b. Dentist
  c. DO
  d. MD

Your Choice: _____

What can you do to figure out what's wrong with this man?

[NEXT PAGE]

You should have this one down pat, by now: Get a Good History. Elicit as much information has you can from the woman who will soon be a widow if you fail.

Through thorough questioning, you find out that the Farmer was in fairly good health until very recently. He hasn't been bitten by any Zombies that she knows of (phew!) He did start complaining a few days ago of some low abdominal discomfort. Nothing severe, just a little annoying. He'd been complaining that he had to pee a lot but, then, he's 75 years old and like all older men, his wife notes, he always peed a lot.

Two days ago, he started losing his appetite and didn't feel like drinking much. She tried to force him to drink more, but he got annoyed and said he had to work. Just yesterday, she found him wandering aimlessly behind the barn. He was unfocussed and couldn't seem to answer any of her questions. She finally got him back to the house and into bed, but he kept trying to get up and wander off, so she tied him down.

Here's a list of SOME POSSIBLE CAUSES for his condition:
1. Stroke
2. Early Zombie infection
3. Urinary tract infection
4. Meningitis (inflammation of the coverings around the brain)
5. Encephalopathy (inflammation of the brain, itself) such as that caused by West Nile Virus
6. Pneumonia

Which do you think is the likely cause?
1. Stroke
2. Early Zombie infection
3. Urinary tract infection
4. Meningitis (inflammation of the coverings around the brain)
5. Encephalopathy (inflammation of the brain, itself) such as that caused by West Nile Virus
6. Pneumonia

Your Choice: _____

How will you figure out which of these causes is correct?

[Next Page]

Aw, c'mon, now: you know it's a physical examination!

The Farmer's skin is thin and dry as is his mouth. His lips are cracked.

Your physical examination shows that he has no fever. His pupils are the same size and equally reactive to light. His reflexes are all normal. He appears to be moving all of his limbs spontaneously.

When you snap your fingers next to his ear, he turns his head to look – and it works equally well on either side.

When you lift his head, his neck bends easily and it doesn't seem to hurt.

There are no bite marks.

His lungs are clear when you listen to them with a stethoscope.

His abdomen is slightly growly, but nothing out of the ordinary.

When you push on his abdomen, as you go further down toward the pelvis, he winces and makes angry faces. When you lightly punch his back, he doesn't seem to react.

What do all these findings tell you?

[NEXT PAGE]

DC:
> If you're a chiropractor, you may recognize the findings or you may not. It pretty much depends on which school you went to.

MD who relies heavily on technology:
> If you're an MD who relies heavily on lab tests to make your diagnoses, this could still present a little problem for you.

DO - or a good MD:
> A good MD or DO, however, should be able to tell what is likely happening.

The Farmer's lungs are clear, so he doesn't have pneumonia.

His neck bends easily and without pain, so it's not likely to be meningitis. Meningitis usually causes a very painful, stiff neck.

Likewise, some kinds of stroke can cause neck pain. Many strokes, however, cause what are called 'lateralizing signs'. If a stroke affects the motor system in the brain (which controls muscle movement) one side of the body would likely show signs of weakness. Some strokes, of course, could just cause disorientation and inability to express one's self, so this remains a possibility.

Encephalopathy (brain inflammation) could, likewise, cause similar symptoms. When the brain swells, however, sometimes problems such as the eyes being unable to move properly or the pupils becoming different sizes, or hearing loss can occur.

It looks to you like an infectious process, but he has no fever.

Hmmm.

Oh, yeah! When you push on his abdomen, it doesn't bother him until you get way down near his pelvis.

You recall your hostess stating that her husband complained that he had to urinate more than usual and then he lost his interest in eating or drinking.

Unfortunately, you can't run any lab tests, so you have to go with your clinical impression.

What's your diagnosis?

[NEXT PAGE]

The farmer has a urinary tract infection.

Even though he has no fever, you're pretty sure. All of his symptoms fit.

In the elderly, two things are more common than in the young: First, they don't develop fevers as readily. Second, even minor infections, like a urinary tract infection, has been known to cause severe disorientation in the elderly, but this usually completely resolves with proper treatment. Such infections can also cause a loss of appetite.

In addition, this man is severely dehydrated which is likely contributing to his delirium.

You don't think the infection has reached his kidneys because usually, when the kidneys become involved, they become inflamed and sensitive. If the kidneys were involved, he would have shown some signs of pain when you hammered on his back just as he did when you pushed on his bladder.

What do you do for him?

DC:
>If you just practice chiropractic, not much.

DO or MD:
>An MD or DO would likely start an IV to hydrate the patient (you have IV equipment in your pilfered supplies). That will help with his strength and might even be enough to reduce the disorientation.
>
>Next, you start the patient on the Bactrim (antibiotic) from your supply, if he's not allergic to it. This should eradicate most simple urinary tract infections.
>
>You've SAVED THE FARMER! ... and maybe all of your lives.

REAL LIFE:

I'm afraid this next example reflects poorly on the medical profession as a whole, but it is a true tale.

While I was in training, I worked in a hospital in Florida. The picture of an aging population inhabiting the entire state isn't quite accurate, but there is, indeed, a disproportionate number of elderly.

While working at the hospital, I had a patient, an older woman who was completely delirious. She was incoherent and had no idea where she was, nor what year it was. Frankly, I thought she'd had a stroke and was about to die. She had all the symptoms our Farmer, above, had.

The sad part is that interns and residents were taking bets on whether or not this 'crazy old lady' would ever leave the hospital, again, or would expire. Honestly, it made me ill to see what the other trainees were doing. I could not take part.

Well, no one actually did the kind of physical exam I described, above. They let the lab tests make the diagnosis for them. Still, her tests showed that she was severely dehydrated and simply had a urinary tract infection. Lo and behold, 2 days later, this lady turned out to be a lovely person, intelligent, and fully cognizant of whom and where she was and ready to go back home – all because she had been hydrated and had her urinary tract infection treated.

"Dammit, Jim, I'm a doctor, not a ….!"

SCENARIO 12

"Ohhh. Owwww. I can't take it, anymore." The smart-aleck teenager is holding the side of his mouth.

The grumpy lawyer is smiling. Payback's a bitch.

You've been watching your adolescent companion for the last few days. He's become more sullen (MORE sullen; he started out sullen … he is a teenager, after all). He's become a lot quieter and less opinionated. (This has had you concerned.) And he hasn't been eating well.

You've asked him if something is wrong but all you ever get is, "No. I'm fine. Quit asking." Of course, that's teen-speak for, "I'll tell you when and if I ever feel like it."

You know you're about to find out the answer.

Grumpy Lawyer: "What's your problem?"

Smart-aleck teenager: "My tooth has been killing me for days. I bit down on that rabbit I'd killed with a shotgun 3 days ago – and bit into a piece of bird-shot. I hurt my tooth. I'd hoped it would go away, but it's killing me."

"Let me take a look," you say. Your teenager grudgingly opens his mouth while you peer inside with a penlight. "I'm not really sure," you say, "But I think the tooth might have a crack."

You feel the jaw. There doesn't seem to be any swelling or sign of infection. There are no pustules or swelling inside the mouth.

Choose your profession:
>   a.   Chiropractor
>   b.   Dentist
>   c.   DO
>   d.   MD

>   Your Choice: _____

What's your next step?
>   [NEXT PAGE]

You wing it. Probably try to pull the tooth and hope it works. Maybe some prophylactic antibiotics (to prevent infection of the tooth socket and jaw).

You should have picked 'Dentist' as your profession for this scenario. What were you thinking??

Section V: WHY YOU SHOULD CHOOSE AN OSTEOPATHIC PHYSICIAN AS YOUR DOCTOR, ESPECIALLY AS YOUR <u>PRIMARY CARE PROVIDER</u>

As stated earlier, this section will answer the question, "If there's so much prejudice and misconception about Osteopathic Medicine, why should I choose an osteopathic doctor and not just an MD, NP, or PA to provide my healthcare?"

If I've done my job well, thus far, the previous section should really have answered much about this concern. Still, for some of you, a few lingering doubts may remain. Here, I will tackle some of the less obvious, but no less important benefits of seeing an osteopathic physician. It should answer any remaining concerns about the basic question, "WIIFM?" (What's In It For Me?)

HOW DOES THIS TRANSLATE INTO THE REAL WORLD?

So far, we have been indulging in a fun, fantasy world where our osteopath is a hero. We can create all the fantastic scenarios we want and imagine our lives in this mythical apocalyptic world, but the question remains, what is the reality of seeing an osteopathic physician for you primary care?

I promised truth in all things, so let me preface this with: not all osteopathic physicians practice medicine osteopathically; many practice allopathically.

The following applies to those osteopathic physicians (and there are still many) who have not succumbed either to the allure of the expedience of allopathic care or to the pressures of managed care (i.e. insurance companies) which push all physicians toward the 5 minute office visit.

1. The Focus of Osteopathic Medicine IS, and ALWAYS
    HAS BEEN, Primary Care

    Osteopathic schools have a history of turning out more
    primary care physicians than allopathic schools by a
    wide margin. Most MD's go into specialty practices
    while most DO's go into some form of primary care.
    This is because, philosophically, Osteopaths are
    oriented toward treating the whole person.

    Since DOs are taught to view the patient as an entire
    being – not just organ systems or disease-tainted parts
    – DO training has always emphasized that a physician
    should care for a patient from top-to-bottom, including
    family issues, emotional issues, and even spiritual
    issues which affect health. The scenarios, above,
    emphasized very specific medical problems and
    demonstrated the problem-solving skills of an
    osteopathic doctor, but more importantly, showed that
    the DO must look beyond the obvious. It is this
    emphasis in our training which makes us particularly
    well-suited as primary care doctors.

    When a patient presents with high blood pressure,
    should we just throw medications at her? Maybe we
    should give her dietary advice? Weight-loss help?
    Talk with the patient to determine whether there are
    behavioral or emotional contributors to the elevation of
    their blood pressure? Delve deeper to find out if there
    are other problems – urinary tract changes which could
    signal kidney injury, which can result in high blood
    pressure?

    All of the above. Our osteopathic training and
    philosophy should direct us to look for the cause of the
    condition, not just a way to mask it by artificially
    lowering the blood pressure. Does that mean we
    wouldn't use medications if that is, in fact, the best

solution? Of course not. We will do what is necessary and what is in the patient's best interest.

How many patients are seen by doctors, every day, who really just throw medicines at them and shoo them out of the office?

Is that the kind of care you want? If not, consider a DO as your primary care doctor.

2. Your well-trained DO will LISTEN to you and TALK with you.

How many times have you gone to a doctor and felt he never really heard a word you said? You could see, almost from the first moment he entered the room or from your first sentence, that he had decided what was wrong with you and had his mind made up about what medicine he was going to give you, what tests he was going to order, and how fast he was going to get out of the room and move on to the next patient?

Communication is key. I've already shown you that 85% of all diagnoses can be made by listening to the patient. For that reason, you will find that unlike many other types of practitioners, once your DO enters the room, he will often greet you warmly and with a smile, take a seat, and focus on you. He will listen to what you have to say and ask questions which not only help him learn more about why you have come to see him, about your illness, and how best to help you, but also lets you know that he is truly hearing you.

The science of medicine cures many ailments. This ART of medicine, helps people.

3. The Internet

The Internet is now a part of our everyday reality. Your doctor shouldn't be afraid of self-educated patients. She should embrace such patients.

The internet has made many of the 'mysteries' of medicine available to the general public. Non-physicians now have access to more information than even some of the best-educated and best-trained physicians once had. The public may not know how to utilize that information to best advantage, but they are far more educated and now have the ability to bring new, medically pertinent information to their physicians. They've learned to question physician pronouncements and physician judgment.

This is a double-edged sword. While they have access to more information, much of the time they misunderstand or misuse it. The physician can be vital in helping patients to understand – and thereby take control – of their own health. Unfortunately, many physicians are still threatened by educated patients.

In my opinion, an educated patient has always been my best ally. As an Osteopathic Physician, I am not only FREE to show my humanity, but my osteopathic professional philosophy and educators encourage it! Instead of having to always have the answer, I can say, let me do some research and we'll figure out this problem.

I've worked with many DOs who take this approach and welcome the information. There are times we can learn from our patients. Not all DOs will feel this way but many, if not most, seem to. Many of the newer MDs will also welcome the patient taking the initiative in learning about their ailments and disorders. Many of the older MDs, however, still balk when a patient presents new information. Not only does it take the physician out of her comfort zone (she was not trained to be receptive in the way DOs always have been), but this may interfere with the planned 5-minute visit. If listening to the patient is not planned for – ingrained in the provider, as it is in the osteopathic physician – how will it be received?

Which type of doctor do you want – one easily threatened by your knowledge and involvement or one who is trained from her first days in medical school to encourage and embrace it?

4. Your well-trained DO will not be afraid to touch you in order to provide the best care for your needs.

How many times have you or someone you cared about gone to a doctor and the physician doesn't even listen to your heart or lungs? Do you feel somehow let down? Cheated? Many people do. Osteopathic training reinforces the necessity of not only listening to what the patient has to say but, also, touching which demonstrate caring that is every bit as important to most people as getting the right diagnosis and the right treatment.

If all doctors operate in a physical vacuum – never touching their patients with a sense of certainty and caring, never listening to their patients with real concern and intensity – then doctors would not only be interchangeable with one another, we would be interchangeable with machines.

A well-trained osteopath brings a dimension to the physician-patient relationship which may be missing in other physician-patient relationships. Our willingness to let the patient invest themselves in their own care, whether through researching on the internet or through explaining themselves so that we understand their concerns and not just their disease processes, makes us very special.

5. The way your well-trained DO uses her sense of touch also adds a dimension to patient care missing from MD, NP, or PA care.

   Palpation, the art and science of touching for the purpose of aiding in diagnosis, is part of the training of all medical professions, but the 'touch' (palpatory) training of DO's goes far beyond what any of the other professions ever learns.

   Touch can, of course, be used as an MD might to determine temperature of the skin, whether organs are enlarged, or whether bones are broken. These are obvious to even the most casual examiner who lays her hands on a patient. Touch can, however, be used for far more subtle diagnostics such as finding why a patient hurts, whether bone is 'out of place,' whether tissues are tighter than they should be and are therefore contributing to pain or restricting movement, and much, much more.

   Your osteopathic doctor is trained in this kind of diagnosis. Find one who is well-trained in hands-on diagnosis and treatment and you will find that many diagnoses may be made more easily, more quickly, more accurately, than via 'traditional methods.

6. Medicine has become non-human.

   MD's are taught to rely heavily on technology for diagnoses and have, at least in the past, spent little time on learning about the importance of relationships with patients. Osteopathic physicians, again, have the advantage. We are taught from our first day in medical school to be human, humane, identify with the patient, not with their disease, and to relate to our patients with patience and listening. Physical diagnosis is strongly emphasized as is TOUCHING the patient. Touch is not just for diagnosis. The need for touch is part of the human condition, a part which most people crave. Touch provides reassurance. It reinforces that the doctor cares.

It is also rewarding for the doctor, believe it or not. Touch is therapeutic for both the patient and the doctor and provides a feedback loop of satisfaction and respect your doctor will never achieve through standard MD-style medicine. People NEED this – both patients and doctors – to really feel connected.

Simply put:
- When your doctor takes TIME to LISTEN to you, you respect her.
- When she does hands-on treatment, you bond with her (and she bonds with you).
- When she instantly cures your pain or medical problem with the touch of her hands, you are amazed by her and adore her!

7. Alternatives to osteopathy always lack.

If you go another route – whether chiropractic or allopathic – you will always know that you have received only half the care you should and will need to visit at least one more provider to get 'complete' care. Your osteopathic physician, on the other hand, is special – the cream of the medical crop in knowledge and abilities. He has studied more about the workings of the body than practitioners of either of the other major medical professions. You need never feel like you are receiving less complete care than you deserve.

The saying goes, "If all you have is a hammer, every problem looks like a nail."

If a chiropractor cannot use medicines or surgery, even if he wants to, will he be constrained to find alternatives which he can provide? Although there may be other solutions, what if the best and most direct solution is a medication? Can he prescribe it? No. Will he refer you to someone who can? Maybe. Even in the best-case scenario, you will need to see another healthcare provider, even if it is just to get an antibiotic.

Moreover, I have seen numerous cases in my practice where a patient has been treated by a chiropractor for years – in one case, FORTY YEARS – with no permanent relief of pain. In many such cases, osteopathic diagnosis and manipulation has completely cured these people. Osteopathy incorporates examination and treatment of muscles, connective tissues, and even non-spine skeletal structures which many chiropractors ignore. If your physician ignores or is ignorant of vital components of the body, might they often be missing components crucial to your health and well-being?

Conversely, what if your MD sees you for back pain and the solution could quickly and easily be fixed by hands-on treatment (manipulation) of the spine or ribs. Would he know how to diagnose the problem and treat it with his hands? No. Would he refer you to a chiropractor or DO who might actually be able to fix you? Maybe. Is he likely to subject you to x-rays, MRIs, and medications, none of which may be necessary? Almost certainly. Would your MD's care, then, prolong your recovery? Definitely. If he did not make an appropriate referral, could his care result in permanent muscular, skeletal, or neurologic dysfunction and possibly permanent pain.

You betcha.

Could such problems be avoided by seeing a well-trained, holistically oriented osteopathic physician?

What do you think?

8. You will know that your doctor never has to be a hypocrite.

Yes, a hypocrite.

Your DO would know the value of many types of medical treatment, whether it be allopathic, chiropractic, naturopathic, homeopathic, etc.

For many decades, the American Medical Association, the overseeing body for MD's in the United States refused to acknowledge the legitimacy of manipulative therapies. It was only in 1980, followed by a decade of subsequent lawsuits, that the AMA eliminated the rule which banned MD's from referring patients to chiropractors. The AMA had, in fact, previously referred to chiropractic as an "unscientific cult" and tried to drive the chiropractic profession to extinction. Suddenly, MD's found themselves forced to acknowledge the legitimacy of chiropractic and thus, manipulative medicine.

Many chiropractors, conversely, often feel that all medications including vaccinations, antibiotics, and many surgeries should never be used. For those of you who are up-in-arms over this statement let me assure you of two important facts: first, I am aware that many chiropractors do not feel this way and happily work with both MD's and DO's in a delightfully collaborative manner. Second, I personally know that many chiropractic schools and practitioners believe or purport to believe exactly what I first stated – that no medicines should ever be used.

The irony is that I also know chiropractors who espouse this line of thought and then immediately seek medications when chiropractic, alone, has failed to cure them. Someone extremely close to me used to work as the manager in the office of a chiropractor who put up signs about the evils of vaccinations and antibiotics. When the chiropractor became very ill, however, he immediately sought antibiotic therapy and cough medicines.

Your DO has no constraint on her judgment. She is free to practice medicine as she sees fit, not disparage the work of others, and choose the tools or treatments which best suit any medical situation – including those affecting the health of yourself and your family – without a guilty feeling of hypocrisy.

9. Why aren't more osteopathic physicians practicing hands-on osteopathic diagnosis and manipulative treatment?

   In other words, "If osteopathic medicine as it should be practiced is so fantastic, why don't ALL osteopaths do what they know is right and incorporate osteopathic diagnosis and manipulative medicine into their practices?"

   Our country is in an ethical struggle between American medicine as it is currently practiced and medicine as it should be practiced. (I promised NO political correctness, not even for DO's, so here comes the dirty laundry.)

   The current method of determining payment – instituted by the government and followed by every insurance company – favors the 5 minute patient visit. Its design specifically, though perhaps not intentionally, inhibits the incorporation of manipulative medicine diagnostic and treatment skills into everyday practice. It also tends to preclude sufficient time for any physician to even converse adequately and genuinely with her patients. In fact, it favors the supplanting of physician-patient time with 'mid-level provider' (PA and NP)-patient time which is less expensive, even though their qualifications are substantially less.

In addition, the current system strongly favors the use of technological tests and treatments, especially the rampant over-utilization of medications. This agenda is pushed by Big Pharma and the multi-billion dollar medical device and healthcare industries including hospitals and insurers. Such 'big business' players have little interest in encouraging low-tech solutions and non-medication solutions – but they have all the money. Big Pharma exerts little pressure on chiropractors, but huge influence over allopathic and osteopathic education, which utilize their products.

These factors make it almost an economic imperative to forego a physician's best judgment and selection of treatments in favor of expedient, well-paid-for but often unnecessary and frequently less-beneficial (or even harmful) tests and treatments. Moreover, many DO's desire for 'acceptance' by their allopathic brethren – as well as some very significant educational gaps in osteopathic education and research – overrides osteopathic principles. DO's are, after all, only human.

In this respect both the MD's and chiropractors actually have a substantial advantage over the DO. MD's are unburdened by the extra knowledge an osteopathic physician has. Chiropractors have very restricted practice options and a relatively narrow perspective. Neither will be burdened by this ethical struggle. MD's (and, unfortunately, many DO's who have opted for the MD-style of practice) have the '5 minute visit' perfected. They hand over the task of diagnosis and treatment to technology and pharmaceuticals.

Many, many chiropractors also have the 5 (or 3) minute visit down to a science and can move patients rapidly through their offices. I know of a collective of chiropractors who promote this type of work and of one chiropractor, in particular, whose normal practice is to see between 600 and 700 patients a week. Over a 40 hour work week, that equates to approximately 3 to 3 ½ minutes per patient.

Staying ethical and being the best physician you know how to be is not an easy road to travel. It is also not a way to riches for most; but it is a very personally rewarding path if you can navigate the impediments the modern healthcare industry – and it is an industry, a business, not a service - has put in the way. As a patient, you need to seek out those osteopathic doctors who remain true to the precepts of osteopathic medicine, encourage them to continue, and demand the kind of care you know you deserve.

Section VI: WHY YOU SHOULD CHOOSE AN OSTEOPATHIC PHYSICIAN AS YOUR PAIN SPECIALIST

Pain has many causes. Frankly, some MDs are excellent at treating certain kinds of pain. If, for instance, pain is due to

1. neuropathic disease (permanent injury directly to the nerves)
2. amputation with residual false nerve impulses which result in pain
3. injury or disease of the central nervous system (the brain and spinal cord)

some MDs do a magnificent job providing the newest medicines, the most up-to-date physical interventions, and the most advanced surgeries.

The problem is, most pain doesn't fall into these categories … but most doctors don't know that. As a result, most chronic pain patients are placed in either categories 1 or 3, above. The majority of pain syndromes actually have their origin in malfunctions of the muscular and skeletal systems, including the connective tissues which bind everything in the body together.

Unfortunately many, if not most, MDs
- Are not trained in hands-on diagnosis and treatment
- Lack the understanding of the neuro-musculo-skeletal systems which every DO is trained in from their first day in medical school
- Have never learned of the contributions of fascia (connective tissue) in maintaining painful sensation
- Are unfamiliar with the principle that injured ligaments and tendons both cause and maintain ongoing painful sensation
- Are unaware that pain which is frequently misdiagnosed as 'neurologic' or 'radicular' (due to

injury of spinal nerves) is actually referred pain from damaged ligaments

- Are unfamiliar with specific pain referral patterns from damaged ligaments and tendons
- Do not know a simple, non-surgical method for repairing such ligaments and tendons thus removing the source of pain
- When faced with an unfamiliar pain pattern may ignore the pain simply because they don't understand it
- May ascribe the pain to the patient's depression or mental status (the "It's all in your head" diagnosis) rather than recognizing that the mental status/depression is a **result** of the chronic pain, not a **cause** of the chronic pain

If you go to a DO who is well-trained in osteopathic hands-on diagnosis and manipulative treatment, however, she will be familiar with all of the above and will be far less likely to miss what might actually be a relatively simple diagnosis and treatment. I can't tell you how many times, for instance, I've had patients come in with upper back and neck pain of many months or years duration – treated with TENS Units, narcotics, pain blockers, rhizotomies (surgical or chemical destruction of nerves to block pain), when all they had was a rib dysfunction which was easily fixed with osteopathic manipulation.

In addition, some DO's who practice hands-on osteopathic diagnosis and treatment also practice prolotherapy.

Conversely, a chiropractor, even if she could recognize the cause of pain, often cannot treat it because either medicine is, in fact, required, or prolotherapy is the proper solution – but in most states, chiropractors can neither prescribe medication nor perform injections.

Would you prefer the physician who can't make the diagnosis but will treat you with medications, surgeries, or other interventions you may not need or would you prefer the one who might be able to make the diagnosis, but is prohibited from treating the problem?

I don't know about you, but if I'm in pain – I want the physician who can make the **right diagnosis** and give me the **right treatment**! I want my DO!

It's also vital to understand that your DO can also diagnose and treat the other causes of chronic pain (neuropathic disease, post-amputation pain, and pain due to central nervous system injury) because he has all the diagnostic tools, medications, and treatments available to him that an MD does. If he can't treat you, himself, he'll know when it's appropriate to refer you for the other medical or surgical interventions.

Section VII: LITTLE KNOW BUT VERY COOL FACTS ABOUT OSTEOPATHIC MEDICINE

Match the correct DO with their accomplishments:

A. Chief Medical Officer of the Marine Corps.

B. Deputy Chief Medical Officer and Chief of Space Medicine at NASA

C. First African-American woman to serve as dean of a U.S. medical school and sister of famed singer Diana Ross. (Okay, this is a gimme: she's the only female on the list.)

D. Former Surgeon General of the U.S. Army and Commanding General of Medical Command. A three-star general, this DO was the first osteopathic physician to serve as Surgeon General in any of the U.S. commissioned services. Prior to serving as Surgeon General of the U.S. Army, this doctor was the commander of the Walter Reed Army Medical Center in Washington, D.C.

1. Lt. Gen. Ronald R. Blanck, DO, MC, USA (Ret.)
2. Richard Jadick, DO, MC, USN
3. Rear Admiral Richard R. Jeffries, DO MC USN
4. Edward Yob, DO
5. James Polk, DO, MS, MMM
6. W. Kenneth Riland, D.O. (deceased)
7. Barbara Ross-Lee, DO

E. Doctor of Osteopathic Medicine whose patients included Richard M. Nixon and Nelson A. Rockefeller

F. Personal physician to former President George H.W. Bush and First Lady Barbara Bush during Mr. Bush's term as vice president.

G. Awarded the Bronze Star with a Combat "V" for Valor. While his unit was engaged in battle with insurgents in Fallujah, this DO set up a make-shift emergency room in the middle of the battlefield in order to treat soldiers' injuries quickly to boost their chances of survival. The doctor's experiences were featured in Newsweek and in a book, <u>On Call in Hell.</u>

Matching Answers:

1 – D
2 – G
3 – A
4 – F
5 – B
6 – E
7 – C

Okay, so you weren't supposed to know the answers.
Hopefully, though, this exercise did help you **appreciate that there are no limits to what a DO can do**!

True or False:

1.	Osteopathic physicians are licensed to practice medicine and surgery in all 50 states and are recognized in at least fifty-five other countries.	True False
2.	Graduates of osteopathic medical schools may enter into MD residency programs and graduates of MD schools may enter into DO residency Programs.	True False
3.	Osteopathy was founded by Andrew Taylor Still, an MD.	True False
4.	Dr. Still's major concern was that conventional medicine focused on the treatment of the effects of disease rather than its causes	True False
5.	Osteopathic medicine, almost from its inception, has been warmly embraced by the MD community who viewed it as a welcome addition to the modern practice of medicine.	True False
6.	Mark Twain once spoke to the New York State Assembly in favor of licensing osteopathic doctors in the state.	True False
7.	During WWII, the osteopathic profession was almost destroyed because MD's, who were in control of medical care for American troops, refused to allow DO's to serve as military physicians – until 1966.	True False
8.	In 1962, it became legal for DO's to purchase an MD license or for MD's to purchase a DO license in California.	True False
9.	Currently, experts believe that osteopathic and allopathic medicine are converging so that one cannot be distinguished from the other.	True False

ANSWERS:
1. True.

2. False

   While it is true that osteopathic medical graduates may enter into MD residency programs, the reverse is not true. Allopathic residents so far outnumber osteopathic residents that DO's could virtually be unable to get an osteopathic post-graduate education if MD's are allowed to enter osteopathic residency programs. Some also contend that MD students lack much of the training that DO students receive, including the principles and practice of osteopathic manual medicine and osteopathic holistic philosophy. Although they are equally qualified in most other ways, MD residents are theoretically unqualified for osteopathic residencies which are supposed to incorporate these principles.

3. True.

   Andrew Taylor Still was an MD who recognized that many of the conventional treatments of the day were useless, at best, and could be quite harmful. He began osteopathy with the idea that the body contains everything it needs to remain healthy, but that sometimes the body could use assistance to open the pathways which deliver nutrition, innate pharmaceuticals, and other as yet unknown substances necessary for health. He also recognized that some surgeries were necessary and some medications could be useful.

4. True.

   He had other concerns, as well, including the fact that many of the medications used at that time, such as arsenic, did more harm than good.

5. False.

    Until the mid-twentieth century, the AMA called
    osteopathic medicine a 'cult.' Accordingly, the AMA
    made it unethical for any MD to even associate with a
    DO.

6. True.

    Lore has it that OMT relieved both symptoms of his
    daughter's epilepsy and Mr. Twain's chronic
    bronchitis. When the legislature tried to ban
    osteopaths from becoming licensed, Mr. Twain, much
    to the consternation of the MD's of the New York
    Medical Society, took up the cause.[12]

7. False.

    There is an irony, here. While it is true that the MD's
    made certain that DO's could not serve as military
    physicians until 1966, it was that very act which may
    have contributed to the rise in popularity of the
    osteopathic profession

    While many MD's went off to war, serving our country
    overseas during WWII, DO's remained at home. As a
    result, with fewer MD's available to care for soldiers'
    loved ones back in America, DO's filled in the service
    gap. Women – wives and mothers of our soldiers,
    abroad – had to go to osteopathic physicians for their
    health care ... and liked it. After the war, when the
    serving MD's came home, they found that many of
    their patients did not return to them, but stayed with
    their osteopathic doctors.

8. False... well, partially true:

    DO's could become MD's, but never the reverse.

In 1962, no MD would ever have been considered fit to purchase an osteopathic medical license due to a lack of training in manual diagnostic and treatment skills as well as osteopathic principles and holistic philosophy. DO's, on the other hand, were apparently deemed to be **at least the equals of MD's.**

The AMA spent millions of dollars to get California state Proposal 22 passed, which eliminated the licensing of osteopaths and the practice of osteopathic medicine in California. The AMA, however, then graciously **invited DO's to become MD's**: "By attending a short seminar and paying $65, a doctor of osteopathy (DO) could obtain an MD degree; 86 percent of the DOs in the state [being unable to otherwise practice, legally] chose to do so."[13] A ruling eventually reversed this situation, allowing DO's to once again resume practicing as a DO and not a paper MD.

9. Sadly, this is true.

MD's make up 93% of all physicians in the U.S. while DO's comprise only 7%. Unless a new crop of students enters the osteopathic profession and once again understand the true nature of osteopathic medicine, DO's - much to the detriment of patients - will again be swallowed up by the much, much larger allopathic community.

OTHER, MORE DAZZLING TIDBITS ABOUT OSTEOPATHIC MEDICINE:

I. Because of their training in neurologic and musculoskeletal medicine, DO's make up a disproportionate number of professional sports team doctors. Many Olympic athletic doctors are also osteopathic physicians.

II. <u>C. Everett Koop, MD</u>: the well-known ***Surgeon General of the United States*** under President Ronald Reagan and the man who forced cigarette companies to put rotated health warning labels on cigarette packs also requiring advertising to include the labels, <u>is an avid proponent of osteopathic medicine</u>. Having experienced firsthand the healing power of OMT, Dr. Koop actually wrote the forward to one of the most important osteopathic manipulative medicine books written, <u>Principles of Manual Medicine</u> by Philip Greenman, DO, FAAO.

III. Another huge proponent of osteopathic medicine is Harvard Medical School graduate and famed author, speaker, and integrative medicine physician **Andrew Weil, MD**. Dr. Weil calls himself "a great advocate of osteopathic manipulative technique (OMT)". Dr. Weil, who does research into complementary and alternative medicine and heads the Arizona Center for Integrative Medicine at the University of Arizona, goes on to say that he is especially an advocate "of cranial therapy. I've found it extremely useful," he says, "for a wide range of problems, from headaches to hyperactivity in children, disturbed sleep cycles and asthma."[14]

IV. Unlike allopathic medical schools, osteopathic medical schools have presented **equal opportunities for women and men from their inception**. According to several sources, including <u>The History of Osteopathic Medicine Virtual Museum</u> operated by the American Osteopathic Association), "Dr. A.T. Still was a visionary whose challenges to the status quo extended beyond the practice of medicine. He was a fervent believer in extending opportunities to all and an early supporter of bringing women and minorities into the profession. ...

"Dr. Still commented, "I opened wide the doors of my first school for ladies...Why not elevate our sister's mentality, qualify her to fill all places of trust and honor, place her hand and head with the skilled arts?" Few career paths were open to women at those times. The first class to convene at the American School of Osteopathy (ASO) in 1892-1893 included women."[15]

Section VIII: HELPFUL RESOURCES

Where you can get more information on Osteopathic Medicine:
1. Book: Quotes, Quips, and Odd Little Bits About –
   Osteopathy and Medicine by Mitchell A. Cohn, DO

Description:

Modern M.D. medicine is simultaneously revered, reviled, deadly serious, and humorously lacking. Osteopathic medicine, despite its wonderful holistic philosophy is no different. Osteopathy is subject to the same reverences, revulsions, and humorous observations. The practitioners of every medical discipline are, after all, only human.

This book of osteopathic wisdom and thoughts about medicine, in general, features quotes from some of osteopathy's supporters, champions, and stars such as Andrew Taylor Still, Mark Twain, Andrew Weil, Edgar Cayce, and more.

Although many of the quotes and thoughts are not from osteopathic physicians – nor even from 'physicians' for that matter, they are representative of what the author considers to be the essence of osteopathy – and the foibles of medicine.

- Be inspired
- Get a chuckle
- See the universal hopes of all medical practitioners
- Appreciate the special qualities of osteopathic medicine and its providers

2. www.ItsAllConnected.net

    Description:

    Osteopathy is about seeing relationships. This extends not only to relationships of one body part to another or relationships of the mind and spirit to the body, but beyond. As Dr. Still was a visionary, looking ahead to the relationships between gender and race to health and healthcare, Dr. Mitchell A. Cohn, DO looks at the relationships of our society and surroundings to our physical, mental, spiritual, and financial well-being; to the health of the individual, of societies, of cultures, and of our Earth. Come join us at ItsAllConnected.net to learn more about Osteopathic Medicine, Osteopathic holistic philosophy, and the impact of each aspect of our lives upon the other; it's not just about healthcare. It's about successful living. Take Osteopathy to the next level.

3. www.MedicalRadical.com

    Description:

    Dr. Cohn's take on medical care isn't always in line with Mainstream Medicine and it isn't always popular – but it is always HONEST and FROM THE HEART. MedicalRadical.com dares to tell the truth about healthcare in the United States when others take the party line. As in his books, Dr. Cohn tackles issues not only about medicine, MD's, alternative practitioners, Big Pharma, and the Hospital system, but even about his own osteopathic profession. Facing the truth, however unpopular, is the only way of fixing it.

    Along the way, pick up interesting opinions from other healthcare practitioners, alternative practitioners, and patients like yourself. You may even learn something useful about a disease or disorder, new treatments, and alternative approaches to treatment.

4. The History of Osteopathic Medicine Virtual Museum - history.osteopathic.org/

5. The American Osteopathic Association - www.osteopathic.org/

    a. Find an osteopathic physician in your area
    b. Learn more about the history of osteopathy
    c. Learn more about today's practice of osteopathic medicine

6. The American Academy of Osteopathy - www.academyofosteopathy.org

    This is the group to which many osteopathic physicians who truly practice Osteopathic Manipulative Medicine/ Therapy (OMM/OMT) belong. If you are looking either for a specialist in manipulative medicine or for a family doctor who also practices quite a lot of manipulative medicine, this would be a great place to contact for a referral.

7. Osteopathic Cranial Academy - www.cranialacademy.com

    Cranial manipulation is a very specific, gentle form of hands-on osteopathic treatment. Its adherents find that manipulation of the bones of the skull have body-wide effects. In particular, cranial manipulation is known to have significant positive effects on the brain, especially in children for problems such as ADHD. It is heartily endorsed by such medical luminaries as Harvard educated Integrative Medicine Expert Andrew Weil, M.D.

8. American Academy of Musculoskeletal Medicine - www.aamsm.com and The American Osteopathic Association of Prolotherapy Regenerative Medicine (affiliate of the American Osteopathic Association) - www.acopms.com

   Prolotherapy is a technique used by many osteopathic physicians who practice manipulative medicine as well as by many MD's, to repair and strengthen ligaments and tendons. These connective tissue components of the body are very frequently the source of chronic pain and muscular and skeletal dysfunction. For that reason, prolotherapy is a perfect complement to osteopathic manipulative therapy (OMT). Whereas OMT restores the orientation and function of muscular and skeletal parts of the body, the body will often fail to maintain these improvements of the support systems – the ligaments and tendons – have micro or macro tears which the body has thus far been unable to repair. Prolotherapy encourages the body to heal these injured structures so that the effects of OMT can be maintained.

   Contact the American Academy of Musculoskeletal Medicine or the American Osteopathic Association of Prolotherapy Regenerative Medicine in order to learn more about prolotherapy or to find a physician who provides prolotherapy in your area.

9. **Pain-Free with Prolo**: How Prolotherapy Stops the Hidden Causes of Pain by Mitchell A. Cohn, DO

   Description:

   This booklet explains in plain language
   - How prolotherapy works
   - How it is used to treat the weakened ligaments and tendons which cause pain

- Why it is the perfect complement to Osteopathic Manipulative Therapy (OMT) in enhancing the treatment of chronic pain
- How the combination of OMT and prolotherapy may provide the only permanent solution to some types of chronic pain
- How your physician can determine whether prolotherapy is right for you

10. The Feminine Touch: History of Women in Osteopathic Medicine by Thomas A. Quinn, DO

    Description (from Amazon.com - www.amazon.com/The-Feminine-Touch-Osteopathic-Medicine/dp/1935503138):

    "In 1892, Andrew Taylor Still did the unimaginable when he accepted women and men equally in his newly opened American School of Osteopathy. Thomas Quinn, DO, showcases some of the valiant women who rose above adversity to become osteopathic doctors in those early years, and includes prominent women osteopathic physicians up to the present time. The stories of their fight against the inequality of the sexes in medicine are intertwined with the struggles of osteopathy to be accepted as a valid scientific practice, illuminating the innovative and determined individuals who helped osteopathic medicine develop into the flourishing profession it is today."

11. The works of Irvin Korr, PhD. - http://www.amazon.com/s/?ie=UTF8&keywords=irvin+korr&tag=googhydr-20&index=aps&hvadid=6352029321&hvpos=1t1&hvexid=&hvnetw=g&hvrand=8067372159306119988&hvpone=&hvptwo=&hvqmt=e&ref=pd_sl_82152yfvuc_e

Dr. Korr was a long-time researcher into the physiology and neurobiology underlying the working of osteopathic manipulation (OMT). Dr. Korr's works underscore, with scientific accuracy and research, the efficacy of OMT. For the skeptic or the very scientifically-minded, reading the works of Dr. Korr may answer at least some of your questions about how and why some forms of OMT work.

Section IX: CONCLUSION

Summary of what was covered:
1. 20 of the most common questions and mis-statements about Osteopathic Medicine.
2. The basics of Osteopathic Medicine including
   a. what osteopathy is
   b. American Osteopathic Medicine vs. non-American Osteopathy
   c. What Osteopathic Manipulative Medicine/Therapy (OMM or OMT) is.
   d. The concept of the Doctor of Osteopathic Medicine as the 'Elite, Complete' physician.
   e. Osteopathic Principles
   f. And SO MUCH MORE!!!
3. Why you should care about osteopathic medicine.
4. Why you want to have an osteopathic physician with you at the end of all civilization.
5. Why you want an osteopathic physician to be your doctor – even if the world doesn't come to an end.

Now, that you have completed reading this book, you
1. Know more about osteopathic medicine than 95% of the U.S. population.
2. You should have a significant idea of what is missing from standard allopathic (MD) education which is taught to virtually all osteopathic medical (DO) students.
3. You should know that in some significant situations, that lack of knowledge could someday put you at unneeded risk of discomfort, poor health, and even worse consequences – and that with proper osteopathic care, you may be able to avoid those situations.
4. You now know that osteopathic hands-on diagnosis and treatment exists and can be a powerful addition to your healthcare.

5. Because of this knowledge you are, at the very least, more likely to choose to visit an appropriate DO, should the need arise.
6. You have learned how to avoid the traps of Big Pharma – the control of medicine and your future medical care by powerful drug companies - and Corporate Medicine:
    a. you have a broader view of health and healthcare than before
    b. a strong understanding of the philosophy that guides your osteopathic physician – which is missing from your MD's education
    c. an understanding that modern technologies and medications are only 2 of the tools in the very large tool chest of diagnostic and therapeutic options available to the well-trained osteopathic physician.
7. You now have a number of resources to learn more about osteopathic medicine, in depth, and to help you decide whether osteopathic medical care is the right path for you.
8. You now also have resources, as well as some helpful hints, about how to find osteopathic physicians, especially those who practice hands-on diagnostics and treatment.

Section X: NEXT STEPS

You have two options:

1. If you're not yet convinced that osteopathic medicine is the right path for you, but you're interested in learning more, I would start your research as soon as possible.

   I recommend, strongly, that you get to personally know a practicing osteopathic primary care physician, as soon as possible: utilize the advice in Section VIII to accomplish this more easily.

2. If you're thoroughly convinced by my snappy prose that Osteopathic Medicine is definitely the right kind of healthcare for you:

   a. Use the resources in section VIII to locate one or more local osteopathic doctors and find at least one with whom you really relate. Not all doctors – not even osteopathic ones – are created equal. Check online ratings for the doctors. Call and have an appointment with them to see if they are someone you'd like to work with.

   b. If you are located in Michigan or are willing to travel to Michigan for treatment of your Severe and Chronic Pain issues, feel free to contact Dr. Cohn. Contact information is provided on the last page of this book.

   c. It's never too early to start to cultivate good relationships with an excellent osteopathic physician. If you already have medical concerns you would like addressed, now is the time to begin you new and better healthcare. If you have no specific concerns, now is the time to begin seeking preventive healthcare counseling and maintenance.

3. BONUSES!!

    a. Finally, if you want to understand how Osteopathic philosophy is more about a way of looking at life and the world we live in and not just a way of looking at the body or even at 'healthcare,' check out my website, www.ItsAllConnected.net for some revealing information and learn what it means when we say, "It's All Connected!"

    b. Check out www.MedicalRadical.com for a doctor's candid view of healthcare, today – the way it is and the way it should be.

*** END ***

Table 1: Scope of Practice: [If scope of practice is likely to be limited: by training, by law in any jurisdictions, or by agreement with a supervising physician, the cell is left empty.]

	DO	MD	NP	PA	DC
Order radiologic tests	√	√	√	√	√
Order lab tests	√	√	√	√	√
Interpret Lab Tests	√	√	√	√	√
Obtain complete medical histories	√	√	√	√	√
Practice medicine without supervision	√	√	√		√
Perform complete physical examinations	√	√	√	√	
Diagnose Acute and Chronic Illness (not limited to neurologic or musculoskeletal)	√	√	√	√	
Treat illness (not limited to neurologic or musculoskeletal)	√	√	√	√	
Prescribe Medication	√	√	√	√	
Perform minor surgery	√	√	√	√	
Perform major surgery	√	√			
Obstetrics	√	√			
Unlimited Scope of medical practice in every state	√	√			
Perform palpatory (touch) diagnosis of significant and also subtle musculoskeletal dysfunction	√	*	*	*	√
Perform spinal manipulation	√				√
Perform musculoskeletal manipulation of all parts of the body	√				
Have an overall holistic philosophy of healthcare and disease prevention	√				√

*Extreme limitations in ability to diagnose musculoskeletal dysfunction via palpation. Limited to only gross abnormalities and generally without ability to diagnose (without technological intervention) or to treat modest or subtle dysfunctions without medication or surgery.

168

DO – Doctor of Osteopathic Medicine (osteopathic physician

MD – Medical Doctor (allopathic physician)

DC – Doctor of Chiropractic (chiropractor)

NP – Nurse Practitioner

PA – Physician's Assistant

GLOSSARY

ALLOPATH:

Medical Doctor; MD. Licensed physician who practices primarily Conventional Western Medicine [See Allopathy, below]

ALLOPATHIC-STYLE MEDICINE:

Allopathy [See below]. A term used when osteopathic physicians practice primarily Conventional Western Medicine without the use of osteopathic manipulation and often without the application of Osteopathic Philosophy [See below]

ALLOPATHY:

1. Conventional Western Medical care as practiced by most MD's.
2. "A system of medical practice that aims to combat disease by use of remedies (as drugs or surgery) producing effects different from or incompatible with those produced by the disease being treated" [Merriam-Webster Dictionary]

CHIROPRACTIC:

"A [system of] health care ... that focuses on disorders of the musculoskeletal system and the nervous system, and the effects of these disorders on general health. Chiropractic care is used most often to treat neuromusculoskeletal complaints, including but not limited to back pain, neck pain, pain in the joints of the arms or legs, and headaches."[16]

CHIROPRACTOR:

Doctors of Chiropractic – often referred to as chiropractors or chiropractic physicians – practice a drug-free, hands-on approach to health care that includes patient examination, diagnosis and treatment. Chiropractors have broad diagnostic skills and are also trained to recommend therapeutic and rehabilitative exercises, as well as to provide nutritional, dietary and lifestyle counseling.

DC:

Chiropractor [See above] DO: Doctor of Osteopathic Medicine [See below]

DOCTOR OF OSTEOPATHIC MEDICINE:

Fully licensed physician and surgeon in the United States; license to practice the unlimited full scope of medicine in all 50 states and all military service branches. A Doctor or Osteopathic Medicine must have received his or her training from one of the accredited osteopathic medical schools in the United States. In addition to learning everything MD's learn and being able to do everything MD's can do – including performing diagnostics, prescribing medications, and performing surgeries - Doctors of Osteopathic Medicine also learn Osteopathic Principles and Philosophy [See below] and Osteopathic Manipulative Medicine. [See below]

MD:

Allopath [See above]

NP:

Nurse Practitioner [See below]

NURSE PRACTITIONER:

"Nurse Practitioners are licensed independent practitioners who practice in ambulatory, acute and long term care as primary and/or specialty care providers. ... In addition to diagnosing and managing acute episodic and chronic illnesses, nurse practitioners emphasize health promotion and disease prevention. Services include, but are not limited to ordering, conducting, supervising, and interpreting diagnostic and laboratory tests, and prescription of pharmacologic agents and non pharmacologic therapies...." [17] It should be noted that Nurse Practitioners are restricted from practicing the full scope of medicine, including surgeries, and may even be restricted from prescribing certain types of medications (narcotic pain relievers, for example) or any medications (in many jurisdictions) without a physician co-signing each prescription.

OMM:
Osteopathic Manipulative Medicine [See below]

OMT:
Osteopathic Manipulative Therapy or Osteopathic Manipulative Therapy [See below]

OSTEOPATH (ah'-stee-oh-path)
1. Osteopathic Physician; Doctor of Osteopathic Medicine; DO. [United States]
2. Non-physician healthcare practitioner who utilizes osteopathic manual (hands-on) diagnosis and treatment as his or her primary form of healthcare practice. Unlike American osteopathic physicians, they are not licensed to prescribe medications or perform surgeries.

OSTEOPATHIC MANIPULATION:
The application of specific positioning and specific forces to specific body parts to effect improvement of bodily function. The purpose is to remove impediments and improve flow of blood and lymphatic fluid as well as neural transmission. This allows freer communication between body parts, organs, and organ systems. Improved communication enhances the flow of neural information as well as better influx of nutrition to - and waste removal from - affected body parts. In addition, the body's inherent pharmacological chemicals from cytokines to hormones flow more freely to and from affected body parts. The overall process is thought to unfetter the body's ability to heal itself.

Unlike Chiropractic [See above], Osteopathic Manipulation is integrated into a broader form of medical diagnostics and therapeutics and includes manipulation not only of the spine, but of any and all affected body parts whose function may be improved by the application of appropriate manipulative techniques.

OSTEOPATHIC MANIPULATIVE MEDICINE:
Application of osteopathic principles [See below] and osteopathic manipulation [See above] to a person after palpatory [see below] diagnosis of neurologic or musculoskeletal abnormalities likely to respond to such manual treatment.

OSTEOPATHIC MANIPULATIVE THERAPY:
Osteopathic Manipulative Medicine [See above]

OSTEOPATHIC MANIPULATIVE TREATMENT:
Osteopathic Manipulative Medicine [See above]

OSTEOPATHIC PHILOSOPHY/PRINCIPLES [2]
1. The body is completely united; the person is a fully integrated being of body, mind and spirit.

   No single part of the body functions independently. Each separate part is interconnected with all others and serves to benefit the collective whole of the person. Alterations in any part of the system, including an individual's mental and spiritual health, affect the function of the body as a whole and all other parts therein.

2. The body is capable of self-regulation, self-healing, and health-maintenance.

   Health is the natural state of the body, and the body possesses complex, homeostatic, self-regulatory mechanisms that it uses to heal itself from injury. In times of disease, when a part of the body is functioning sub-optimally, other parts of the body come out of their natural state of health in order to compensate for the dysfunction. During this compensatory process, however, new dysfunctions may arise. Osteopathic physicians must work to adjust the body so as to realign its parts back to normal. Osteopathic manipulative medicine aims to restore the body's self-healing capacity by decreasing allostatic load, or the physiologic effects of chronic bodily stresses,1 and enhancing the immune system.

3. Structure and function are reciprocally interrelated.

    The structure of a body part governs its function, and thus abnormal structure manifests as dysfunction. Function also governs structure. In addition, if the body's overall structure is suboptimal, its functioning and capacity for self-healing will be inhibited as well.
4. Rational treatment is based on an understanding of these three aforementioned principles.

    These basic osteopathic tenets permeate all aspects of health maintenance and disease prevention and treatment. The osteopathic physician examines, diagnoses, and treats patients according to these principles.

OSTEOPATHY (ah-stee-ah'-puh-thee)
1. [United States] the artful and scientific practice of medicine incorporating Osteopathic philosophy [See above] as well as osteopathic manipulative medicine [See above], and all western conventional medicine [See Allopathy, above] including the use of all good and proper and scientifically valid technologies, diagnostic techniques, pharmacologic and surgical treatments. Osteopathy also tends to emphasize health optimization and disease prevention.
2. [Countries other than the United States] A form of healthcare practice which incorporates all of the tenets

and principles of Osteopathic philosophy and osteopathic manipulative medicine, but without the incorporation of most western technologies, diagnostic techniques, or pharmacologic or surgical treatments. Practitioners of this limited form of Osteopathy are usually not considered 'physicians' within their countries of practice and are not licensed as such in those countries.

PALPATION:
Using the sense of touch to diagnose malfunctions within the body.

PA:
Physician's Assistant [See below]

PHYSICIAN ASSISTANT:
"… a medical professional who works as part of a team with a doctor. … [a physician assistant must] practice medicine with the supervision of a physician.[18] Unlike a Nurse Practitioner, a Physician Assistant may never practice independently, without direct physician supervision. A Physician's Assistant's scope of practice is not so much limited by licensure, but by the operating agreement he/she has with his supervising physician.

PT:

Physical Therapist. A member of the Physical Therapy profession who is "concerned with promotion of health, with prevention of physical disabilities, with evaluation and rehabilitation of persons disabled by pain, disease, or injury, and with treatment by physical therapeutic measures as opposed to medical, surgical, or radiologic measures." [19]

Bibliography

[1]Charles D. Ogilvie, "OSTEOPATHIC MEDICINE,"
Handbook of Texas Online
(http://www.tshaonline.org/handbook/online/articles/sdo01).
Published by the Texas State Historical Association.

[2]Patrick Wu and Jonathan Siu, A Brief Guide to Osteopathic
Medicine For Students, By Students
(http://www.aacom.org/resources/bookstore/Documents/Brief-
Guide-to-OME_Final.pdf). Published by the American
Osteopathic Association.

[3]Quote from Wikipedia: source material: Ronald H. Cole,
1997, *Operation Urgent Fury: The Planning and Execution of
Joint Operations in Grenada 12 October – 2 November 1983*.
Joint History Office of the Chairman of the Joint Chiefs of
Staff Washington, DC

[4]Quote from Wikipedia: original source - R. P. Turco, O. B.
Toon, T. P. Ackerman, J. B. Pollack, and Carl Sagan (23
December 1983)."Nuclear Winter: Global Consequences of
Multiple Nuclear Explosions". Science 222 (4630): 1283–92.

[5]Spine (Phila Pa 1976). 2007 Oct 1;32(21):2375-8; discussion
2379. Safety of chiropractic manipulation of the cervical spine:
a prospective national survey. Thiel HW, Bolton JE, Docherty
S, Portlock JC.

[6]Spine (Phila Pa 1976). 2007 Oct 1;32(21):2375-8; discussion
2379. Safety of chiropractic manipulation of the cervical
spine: a prospective national survey. Thiel HW, Bolton JE,
Docherty S, Portlock JC.

[7]J Manipulative Physiol Ther. 2004 Mar-Apr;27(3):197-210.
Safety of spinal manipulation in the treatment of lumbar disk

herniations: a systematic review and risk assessment. Oliphant D. [LUMBAR]

[8]JAMA. 2010;303(13):1259-1265. Trends, Major Medical Complications, and Charges Associated With Surgery for Lumbar Spinal Stenosis in Older Adults. Richard A. Deyo, MD, MPH; Sohail K. Mirza, MD, MPH; Brook I. Martin, MPH; William Kreuter, MPA; David C. Goodman, MD, MS; Jeffrey G. Jarvik, MD, MPH

[9]With many thanks to the Zombie Research Society ... yes, it really exists!: http://zombieresearchsociety.com

[10] Alien Apocalypse: 2005 Sci-Fi Channel made for TV movie, written by Josh Becker (credited) and Robert Tapert (uncredited). Directed by Josh Becker. Starring Bruce Campbell and Renee O'Connor. http://www.beckerfilms.com/AlienApocalypse-p1.htm

[11]Harold I. Magoun Jr, DO, FAAO, FCA, DO ED (Hon), "More About the Use of OMT During Influenza Epidemics," Journal of the American Osteopathic Association, J Am Osteopath Assoc October 1, 2004; vol. 104 no. 10 406-407.

[12]"MARK TWAIN, OSTEOPATH," *The New York Times*, February 28, 1901

[13]Howell, J. D. (1999). "The Paradox of Osteopathy". New England Journal of Medicine 341 (19): 1465–1468.

[14]See Dr. Weil's blog: http://www.drweil.com/drw/u/id/QAA269342

[15]The History of Osteopathic Medicine Virtual Museum website: http://history.osteopathic.org/

[16]"What Is Chiropractic?" American Chiropractic Association website: http://www.acatoday.org/level2_css.cfm?T1ID=13&T2ID=61

[17]"What Is A Nurse Practitioner?" Frequently Asked Questions, American Academy of Nurse Practitioners. http://www.aanp.org/NR/rdonlyres/A1D9B4BD-AC5E-45BF-9EB0-DEFCA1123204/4710/2011FAQswhatisanNPupdated.pdf

[18] American Academy of Physician Assistants (AAPA)

[19] Stedman's Medical Dictionary 28th Edition, 2006. Published by Lippincott Williams & Wilkins.

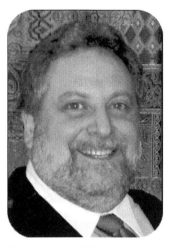 **Dr. Mitchell A. Cohn, DO**
received his undergraduate
degree from the University of
Michigan, Ann Arbor, in 1981.
In 1986, he received his Doctor
of Osteopathic Medicine degree
from the University of
Osteopathic Medicine and Health
Sciences in Des Moines, Iowa.
Dr. Cohn went on to do a
traditional osteopathic internship
at the Community Health Center
of Branch County, Coldwater,
Michigan – a Michigan State
University-affiliated program. He subsequently received post-
graduate training in Family Medicine and
Biomechanics/Osteopathic Manipulative Medicine through
programs at Michigan State University, as well.

For much of his career, Dr. Cohn has been in a solo private
practice in general medicine with special interests in the field
of Osteopathic Manipulative Medicine and the treatment of
pain and neurologic and musculoskeletal injury. He was also
the founder and chief medical legal consultant for 2 legal
medicine consulting firms. He is also an award-winning author
and has had his work published in professional journals.

In addition to typical osteopathic medical training, Dr. Cohn
has extensive knowledge and expertise in hands-on
manipulative treatment and evaluation. He also places a great
deal of emphasis on finding and treating the very subtle and
often gradual changes in a person's body which can lead to
great pain and dysfunction. He emphasizes finding the root
problem from which a person's pain or health problem stems,
rather than just treating the symptoms.

Dr. Cohn has experienced a great deal of success in treating
acute and chronic pain such as headaches, neck pain, upper and
lower back pain, TMJ problems, musculoskeletal chest pain,

chest-wall pain, post-surgical chest pain, failed-back syndrome (post-laminectomy or discectomy pain), and even structurally-induced neuropathic and radicular pain of the limbs.

Dr. Cohn is also the author of numerous short stories including "Home-Sick" and the well-received "Misplaced Messiah," as well as a book on parenting, Common Sense Parenting - Raising Extraordinary Kids by using the Golden Rule and Other Simple Concepts (For Ages 2 and Up), and the Osteopathy and the Zombie Apocalypse books for pre-medical/pre-college students and for laypeople.

Dr. Cohn speaks to general audiences; high school, college and pre-medical students, and pain patients introducing them to Osteopathic Medicine, principles, and practice. He also speaks to osteopathic medical students to broaden their understanding of the applicability of hands-on medicine to modern medical practice and to deepen their appreciation for the advantages hands-on diagnostics and treatment can provide in this world of over-reliance on medical technology. He works to enlighten patients, doctors, and other medical personnel about osteopathic medicine, in general, to encourage students to investigate osteopathy as a career choice, and to inform patients about alternative treatments, especially for chronic pain.

CONTACT DR. COHN:

FEEDBACK IS WELCOME!

- Please email any **feedback, comments, or questions** regarding this book to: **Dr.MACohn@ItsAllConnected.net** or **Dr.MACohn@MedicalRadical.com**

- Inquiries regarding engaging Dr. Cohn for **SPEAKING** at your event may be sent to either of the above emails or to: **Dr.MACohn@hotmail.com** or via **fax** at **+1(517)798-5029**

- Inquiries regarding engaging Dr. Cohn to **consult about treatment** of pain or other health problems may be sent to Dr. Cohn via **fax** at **+1(517)798-5029**

- You may also reach Dr. Cohn via **telephone** at **+1(517)376-3228**

Please, visit our websites:
www.ItsAllConnected.net
and
www.MedicalRadical.com

Made in the USA
Charleston, SC
27 February 2013